Also by
Robert M. Duggan

Common Sense for the Healing Arts

Robert M. Duggan

Breaking the Iron Triangle

Reducing Health-care Costs in Corporate America

WisdomWell Press
Columbia, Maryland

BREAKING THE IRON TRIANGLE:
Reducing Health-care Costs in Corporate America

Copyright © 2012, Robert M. Duggan

Published by WisdomWell Press
www.wisdomwellpress.com

WisdomWell Press
8955 Guilford Road, Suite 240
Columbia, MD 21046

Printed in the United States of America
Signature Book Printing, www.sbpbooks.com
Book design: David M. Buscher
Cover design: Human Mvmnt, LLC

First Edition

10 9 8 7 6 5 4 3 2 1

Library of Congress Control Number: 2012936753

ISBN
Hardcover: 978-0-9856352-0-6
Softcover: 978-0-9856352-2-0
Ebook: 978-0-9856352-1-3

THE IRON TRIANGLE
Our National Health-care Conundrum

COST

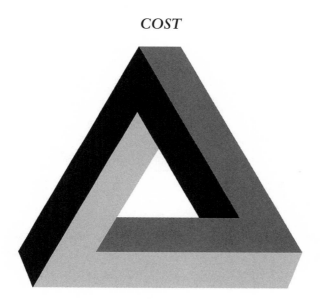

ACCESS   *QUALITY*

Cutting *Costs* means rationing *Access* or reducing *Quality*.
IMPOSSIBLE

Increasing *Access* to the uninsured means increasing *Costs* or
reducing *Quality*.
IMPOSSIBLE

Increasing *Quality* means adding *Costs* or rationing *Access*
IMPOSSIBLE

What is possible for us as a nation?

I dedicate these essays to two individuals who inspire me to live from love and from friendship:

Ivan, who taught me to think, and Susan, who taught me to love.

Together, they taught me to serve life with conviviality. Their friendship calls me to unify the work of the academy and the work of the heart.

And to my grandchildren, who remind me daily that it is my honor and my duty to pass on through them the wisdom I have received from my ancestors:

Tamar, Lennox, Rianna, Ava, Adrien, Dominick, Maxim, Roman

Thanks to all who made this book possible . . .

In writing these essays, I reflect the gifts of life as they are given to me. Dear reader, you are served by many individuals who have inspired and contributed to the preparation of this book.

These essays are the fruit of more than a year of collaboration with David M. Buscher, who has gently nudged me to clarify and simplify, to shorten and to focus, to eliminate what would have been distracting. To the extent that my writing readily serves your understanding, please thank David. And David's attention to the content has been matched by the devotion to precise detail and language by Mary Ellen Zorbaugh, who has been my writing teacher for more than 30 years. A deep bow of gratitude. These essays would not exist without the flowing collaboration of both of you.

Many individuals carefully read early versions of these essays and offered wonderful comments and encouragement. I am most grateful to Bob Benjamin, Pat Frontera, Guy Hollyday, Karen Howard, Karen Jordan, Greg Kiley, Nancy Lilly, Regina McPhillips, Simon Mills, Deborah Mizeur, Maci Moser, David Schwartz, James Snow, Linnea Varner. In addition, I am grateful to Catherine Baase, Peter Beilenson, Blaize Connelly-Duggan, Jade Connelly-Duggan, Hal Gunn, Nortin Hadler, Wayne Jonas, and Tom Reilly for their attention to detail in particular parts of the manuscript. I bow with gratitude to Joy Andrews, Juliet Farrell, Suzanne Shutty, and

David McKaig for their work in enabling these ideas to move outward into the marketplace of ideas. A special debt of gratitude is due to my dear friend, Ed Stephenson, for his constant support throughout this entire project.

This work is also the result of many years of serious conversations with my colleagues. I especially honor Dianne Connelly, my colleague, friend, and partner of many years and the mother of my children, who has taught me the power and nuance of language, that words are medicine, and that all sickness is really homesickness.

I am grateful for an ongoing dialogue with Nortin Hadler, who has taught me to trust my deep instinct that we humans are able to be well without turning over our power, our lives, and our wellness to experts. And I am grateful for conversations with Simon Mills, conversations that began in 1981 and from which has emerged my clarity about the possibility of restoring to each individual and family the power of self-care.

I doubt I would have been able to listen to the wisdom of my teachers and friends, students and patients if I had not been guided by my life mentor, Ivan Illich, who taught me to listen and question in a unique way. I first met Ivan in 1952 when he was not yet the great historian and scholar but my parish priest, and I was his altar boy. From those first moments he challenged me to question the assumptions upon which my thoughts and opinions were grounded . . . from the beginning he taught me to be aware that everything was based on made-up human assumptions. Any unique perspectives I offer in this book are rooted in his questioning. I am offering this work as mine, not at all claiming it reflects Ivan's perspective. However, I acknowledge that whatever skill I have in opening new perspectives I derive from many hours of conversation in which he questioned and challenged me. Thank you, Ivan, for always reminding me of what matters – friendship, hospitality, and service – and to always question what we hold as certitudes. May you rest in peace.

I honor and thank my grandfather, Mike Whitty, and my father,

Maurice Duggan. I am grateful for the support and encouragement of all my family, particularly my children, Blaize and Jade, and Susan's children, Suzanne and Scott. I see them living wonderful lives for their families and children, passing along hospitality and wisdom to the next generation.

I am especially grateful to my beloved Susan, who has encouraged me to go forward with this work and endured me as I've moved through the process of writing and rewriting. I thank you, Susan, for keeping me on task, for your love, warmth, dignity, courage, and shared commitment to being of service to the next generations. You truly live your promise of being a radiant, loving embrace to all who are in your presence.

GUIDE TO THE ESSAYS

A Word About the Author, *and* How to Read These Essays

When asked, "What thing about humanity surprises you the most?" the Dalai Lama answered: "Man . . . Because he sacrifices his health in order to make money. Then he sacrifices money to recuperate his health. And then he is so anxious about the future that he does not enjoy the present, the result being that he does not live in the present or the future; he lives as if he is never going to die, and then dies having never really lived."
– Although the origin is uncertain, this quote is widely attributed to the Dalai Lama XIV.

A WELL-RESPECTED senior public health officer told me the following story a few years ago. I had known this person professionally for some time, and I knew that as a very traditional public health officer, he was reluctant to support the wellness approach to health care that I advocate. In a personal capacity, however, he had asked me about some family issues regarding pain and disease. I recommended that he and his wife learn yoga. And indeed, they began to do yoga; and he told me how much they enjoyed and benefited from it.

Then one day, home alone, he fell while coming down the stairs. The pain in his back was excruciating, and he felt he could not move. He knew he needed to call 911 but had no way to access a phone. As he lay motionless on the stairwell platform, he had the thought that perhaps some of the breathing techniques he learned in yoga might help. He began to breathe deeply, mainly to settle himself. Then he thought that some of the other things he had learned in yoga also might be helpful. It took about 15 minutes, but after settling down through breathing and then stretching out with yoga techniques, his pain was gone. He got up and walked down the stairs, never calling 911. He was keenly aware that if he had called an ambulance, the expense probably would have been close to three thousand dollars, whereas helping himself with yoga was free.

I'm sad when I think that he did not immediately turn that learning experience into a public health campaign. The resources were available to him, but it would have meant his "coming out of the closet" with a radical approach.

The public continues to be told to dial 911.

Instead, often they first could be told to "breathe."

Bob Duggan's "Health"

With every disease event in my life, from the serious pneumonia my father sweated me through at age seven, I have lived well with only minor medical interventions. Looking back, I am sure I would have been diagnosed as manic-depressive in my twenties and put on lithium for life if I'd had access to a physician. Fortunately, before my cycle of stimulation and collapse became pathological, with the help of friends I was able to determine that my lifestyle was the major factor.

In 1971 when I was 31 years old, my hands and feet came to be in such pain that I could hardly drive a car. I discovered later the pain was a side effect of an over-the-counter medication I'd been given in Hong Kong for diarrhea. That product, a prescription drug in the USA, eventually was removed from the market due to cardiac side effects. When the pain became unbearable, I resorted to treatment by an acupuncturist in England – treatment that was highly and immediately effective. The practitioner, Professor J. R. Worsley, said, "Thank God your body was so wise. Your body protected your heart by restricting the function of your extremities." (At that time, neither of us knew anything about the medication's later-reported side effects.)

His treatment impacted my life, and I stayed in England to study healing. More importantly, his *words* had an even more profound impact. As one trained in philosophy, I immediately understood if his words were correct ("your body is wise"), then modern medical science was based on a false set of assumptions and had become increasingly disconnected from reality since the time of Descartes.

I understood (I remember thinking this outside his clinic after saying goodbye on the third visit) that health care was a way to change modern thought at a most profound level. Health care is the only arena of life that no one, no matter how wealthy, can avoid. It is impossible not to deal with pain and suffering because it affects all individuals and their elders and children. How we deal with pain impacts how we think about life – this was reinforcement of the message I had received from my mentor, Ivan Illich, who in 1973 also was in Oxford researching his classic text, *Medical Nemesis,* in which he essentially says that how a culture thinks about suffering and death determines whether it will spend itself out of existence attempting to avoid both.

My perspective in writing this book arises not only from my personal experience and personal passion, but also from listening to the stories in approximately 30 patient visits every week for the past 40 years. My patients have taught me medicine; they have taught me healing; they have taught me wisdom.

As of this writing, I am 72 years old. This year, 2012, I will pay $5,646 for medical insurance, and my wife will pay an even higher amount. Although I have been eligible for Medicare for seven years, I've never used it for a medical service, except once to pay for physical therapy due to a tightness in my left shoulder. In this aspect, you might say I am not a good American consumer; I'm certainly atypical. At my age more than 60 percent of American males are on three or more prescription drugs.[1] If you are an American taxpayer, my lifestyle has saved you money. Because I consume so few health-care products, the hospital and pharmaceutical companies do not appreciate my lifestyle – my approach to life is dangerous to their business model.

When I chose to focus my life's work on the arena of health care in society, it was not because I was initially interested in health care or in acupuncture, but because, as a philosopher, I questioned some of the basic assumptions of our modern society about life and science and community. No one in society can avoid the issues of pain and suffering and death. We all must deal with these challenges whether we are Republican, Democrat, or Independent; and we all deal with them with great pragmatic urgency. This is where ideology inescapably hits the wall of reality.

How to Read These Essays

Think of reading these essays as an opening to a conversation with me. The thoughts shared in this book grow out of my personal life experience and 40 years of clinical practice, as well as what I've learned in developing professional education programs and working successfully with policy initiatives – such as the experience I gained in the 1970s when I established my right to offer my services as an acupuncturist healer to the community.

When I opened my practice, acupuncture was largely illegal in America. Forty years later, that reality seems strange to many. Today, acupuncture is only one among many low-tech, high-touch healing arts.

It is essential we bring commonsense, low-tech approaches into the mainstream of society, enhancing well-being and cutting wasteful expenditures.

When I say this is "common sense," I do not mean my own made-up "common sense"; rather I am reporting the wisdom spoken by thousands of patients and students over many years, wisdom repeatedly gathered and reexamined in serious classroom and treatment room conversations. What I share is truly the wisdom of patients and many generations of people as I have digested their speaking.

I am aware these essays reflect my perception of the world and the narrative I create for myself, my family, my grandchildren, and my students. I ask you to be open to noticing how these thoughts resonate with your knowing of the world.

I do not attempt to justify or document many of my perceptions. I do provide references and guides to many of my teachers – individuals who over the many years have enriched my understanding through their writings and speaking; and the figures and calculations on which I base my recommendations are supported by footnotes.

I speak with repetitive patterns and themes. You will find some of my learning/teaching stories repeated in several places for two reasons:

Each time, the story is presented in a different context and brings a different perspective on life. Also, this is a book about a new perspective on many well-worn conversations. After 45 years as a classroom teacher, it is clear to me that the listener/reader absorbs only a small percentage of the message each time. (At my age, I'm very aware that I wish I had listened more fully to my teachers many years ago.) As a teacher, I believe that repetition, repetition, repetition engenders openings to new possibilities and to new understandings and insights.

NOTES

1. National Center for Health Statistics. "Health, United States, 2010." See Table 94. Available at http://www.cdc.gov/nchs/data/hus/hus10. pdf#listtables.

Overview

"In every society the dominant image of death determines the prevalent concept of health."[1]
– *Ivan Illich*

IT HAS BEEN estimated that we can shift more than $1 trillion dollars annually from health-care expenditures to more productive aspects of our national economy; and we can do that by changing the way we think about and tend what are called non-communicable lifestyle diseases such as diabetes, obesity, hypertension, heart disease, cancer, etc., from a high-tech, fear-driven approach to a high-touch, low-tech, commonsense wellness approach.[2] These essays point to ways of thinking, speaking, and acting I assert are essential to redirecting the use of these funds to more enjoyable aspects of living – and frankly, to avoid the financial bankruptcy that confronts our nation because of uncontrolled medical expenditures.

As a nation we must turn the medical conversation away from a war on disease and fear of our bodies, and expand our focus on learning and understanding ways of living well, being of service and enjoying life. It is in this context that I hold this entire book.

The first essays – Part One, "The Crisis" – challenge powerful fundamental assumptions embedded in our culture which, while deeply cherished, demonstrably do not serve our personal or national interests. We point out these assumptions and then, in sequence, explore their impact and look at what must be done to begin to shift them, asking new and different questions, for example: What would it be like if we started from a clean slate to generate wellness for our national community? Then we examine many of the firm linguistic constructs flowing from these assumptions – constructs, I say, we use repetitively and do not provide a way for change.

In subsequent essays we look at the stark data that confirm our crisis situation. In the essay titled "Economics 101," we explore the current economics of health care and why the existing economic conversation about health care is not feasible and indeed, is truly calamitous.

These first essays also examine the conundrum of cost-quality-access, a triangle that has been impossible to break because it focuses on a wrong-headed set of assumptions. This "iron triangle" is unbreakable if health care is thought about in terms of a high-tech intervention in a battle with death and disease. When this triangle is examined in light of low-tech interventions already in place in many corporations and government projects, it proves to be a false conundrum.

The last essays illustrate a new perspective on American health care, a model for moving forward. They point to many components of a wellness system already in place on a small scale across America. These essays build on different assumptions and on research pointing in a creative direction. "Economics 101" shows how, together, we can create a new economics for health care.

These essays conclude with specific proposals that can be implemented at no cost to the taxpayer, and indeed offer the possibility of significant savings to the taxpayer as well as profits to private investors.

These initiatives will make an enormous difference for the world of our grandchildren:

- *Encourage entrepreneurial demonstrations in corporations and government health-care programs which, by enhancing the wellness of our citizens, avoid many existing costly medical interventions.*

- *Deliver such programming to our school teachers as part of their employee benefits, thus reducing the medical costs of their employment and, perhaps more importantly, have a beneficial spillover effect on parents and children.*

- *Deliver wellness programming to our military families, troops, and veterans, with the same spillover effect on our society as a whole.*

- *Design health stat systems to enable the delivery of low-cost, low-tech care to the specific individuals who are costing the system the most.*

All of these interventions will be more than self-funding through proven cost savings. In fact, they are attractive to entrepreneurs as profitable investments.

This is a commonsense approach that restores to American citizens the right to be their own primary care provider – a privilege and a right that has been suppressed by epic turf battling among professional groups and by the disempowering custom in our culture (and economy) of turning our bodies over to specialists who ignore or overrule our natural instinct for wellness.

In proposing to change health care as we know it in the USA, I am dealing with changing the basic assumptions of 17 percent of our national GDP, and with a financial arena that is growing significantly into a higher percentage of our GDP. With burgeoning medical costs and the desire to reduce these costs, health care might be an arena in which it is possible to divert the common gaze from the accumulation of material goods to the accumulation of common sense and the wider common good. I believe these qualities of common sense and a focus on the common good have a higher value in economies that have exceptional health-care outcomes. And it can be achieved at a fraction of the costs.

After 40 years of surviving as an acupuncturist on the edge of the existing health-care industry, I am not naïve. I realize it is immensely difficult to create significant change in the world of health care. The pharmaceutical industry, the hospital industry, the medical industry – these are entrenched, very powerful forces that have a large economic stake in the current movement of health care and the rising costs of health care.

I do not propose fighting with any aspect of that industry. I have benefited from it. My leg was repaired by surgery, and I have survived infections because of antibiotics. Together, all of us have invented this world with our desire for the magic quick fix for our pains. This is fine and often serves well. Today we, the American public, are simply asking this medical system, with all of its related industries and interests, to accomplish things it was never designed to do. The system is marvelous with disease, yet *it is not designed to make us live wisely and thus avoid disease in the first place.*

These commonsense essays point to ways to minimize the use of this high-tech, high-cost system and to allow it, over time, to organically "right-size" itself.

At the same time, these essays point to ways of greater personal enjoyment and empowerment, to moving away from fear of life toward real-time benefits of "right living."

I offer this writing as a contribution to a critical public conversation I often experience as a conversation near the edge of despair.

Dear reader, before you continue, I ask your deep listening and your open-minded attention. This book offers a different perspective; and thus I request a suspension of your current beliefs, any quick judgments, or even, perhaps, of any cynicism. Please let go of your formed conclusions and allow for a slow ripening of ideas you may find useful.

A great deal is at stake for all of us.
Blessings.

Bob Duggan
Columbia, Maryland
Spring 2012

Part One: The Crisis
Essay 1 – We ("We," the American public) are operating with a set of cherished and destructive assumptions.
Essay 2 – As a result, we are asking the wrong questions.
Essay 3 – We notice that we have a health-care monopoly.
Essay 4 – We review the current monopoly as a disaster for America.
Essay 5 – We look at language and ideas that do not serve.
Essay 6 – We ask whether our bodies are smart or dumb.
Essay 7 – We look at an economics of health care that is not working.

Part Two: The Opportunity
Essay 8 – We look at a set of useful assumptions.
Essay 9 – We look at examples of thriving communities.
Essay 10 – We look at a workable economics.
Essay 11 – Entrepreneurial Actions: Recommendations that have no cost to the taxpayer and potential huge returns on investment.

NOTES

1. Ivan Illich, *Limits to Medicine: Medical Nemesis, The Expropriation of Health* (Marion Boyars Publishers, 2000, p. 74).

2. Ross DeVol and Armen Bedroussian, "An Unhealthy America: The Economic Burden of Chronic Disease. Charting a New Course to Save Lives and Increase Productivity and Economic Growth." (Milken Institute Executive Summary and Research Findings, October 2007). Available at www.milkeninstitute.org.

Part One: The Crisis

Four Cherished *and* Destructive Assumptions

"I'm better in myself. Oh, yes, I still have my pains,
but they don't bother me anymore."
– A patient, in response to the question, "How are you?"

I HAVE BEEN tending people as a health-care provider, a teacher, a mentor for over four decades. I am an acupuncturist; acupuncture is the core skill I use and am licensed to practice. However, what I do day to day is largely listen, question, observe, and teach. The longer I do this, the more I am aware the core teaching is often as simple as: "Please, take a deep breath. Please, get more sleep. Please, drink more water. Please, go for a walk." More often, the core exercise that enables better functioning of the mind, body, and spirit is mundane, very obvious, very natural, very basic, very easy for anyone to do.

I've taken seriously the comments made by patients over these 40 years. One of the most basic comments was made early on by a woman in England who repeatedly said things strange to my ears. When I asked, "How are you?" she replied, "I'm better in myself. Oh, yes, I still have my pains, but they don't bother me anymore." That's an extraordinary concept – what is the possibility of us being both well and not bothered by our pains?

I had a similar conversation about 25 years ago with Charlie, a patient who said to me, "You know, I never thought asthma would become my friend. But since I've started acupuncture, I realize I get minor symptoms of asthma long before I get the attack that usually brings me to the emergency room and puts me back on drugs. If I pay attention to those minor symptoms, I find they are alerting me I've not been getting enough sleep, I've been in upset with my family or my work, or I've been having too much caffeine and not eating properly. They alert me to pay attention to my lifestyle. Since I've been doing that and paying attention to the minor asthma symptoms, I've not had a single major incident."

I've been struck by some studies on the effectiveness of acupuncture. A study by Claire Cassidy published in 1997 pointed out patient satisfaction was not correlated with the relief of a person's symptoms. Patient satisfaction in that study was correlated with "I now understand how I generate my symptoms."[1]

Over the years, I've noticed the everyday comments of the people I'm serving raise questions in myself about what I thought I was doing as a "health professional." As I've reflected on those comments, I've come to realize what I thought were the basic assumptions of my work – that I'm there to take responsibility for making people better, getting rid of their diseases, preventing death, alleviating suffering – were perhaps part of a mistaken agenda. Perhaps those assumptions were impossible.

Several years back, I was at the opening of a new public health program at Morgan State University. A panelist at the event said to the audience, "Most of us wouldn't be here if our grandparents were dependent on modern Western medicine. It didn't exist in their lifetime and thus wasn't available to them. And yet, somehow we're here. Maybe we have to recover what our grandparents knew before we get more dependent on modern technology."

Forty years of clinical experience thus led me to question four distinct assumptions. They are assumptions that are widely held by our culture and yet are rarely discussed as operating assumptions for our health-care system. A reexamination of these assumptions in the light of history, in the light of how our ancestors lived, and in the light of the phenomena we live with daily may have a profound impact on public policy.

For each of these assumptions there will be a case – a story – and then a statement of the assumption to be questioned.

Story Number One: Living Fully in the Presence of Death

When I think of our health-care system, I often think about my experience with Larry and Peg about 10 years ago. Larry was a very successful businessman who came to me after he had developed cancer. Larry's family and friends wanted me to help him recover from the cancer. When Larry and I spoke, he had no such illusion. He wanted some more good time that summer to play golf and to live fully in his days before his death. As Larry put it, "I've lived a wonderful life, and I want to go on living fully. I know that I'm going to die."

Late that summer, I received a message and a request: Larry was in the hospital with pneumonia, and would I visit him. I went to visit Larry, took a look, and saw what a physician before 1908 would have called the signum mortis, *the signs of death. This, I thought, was much more serious than pneumonia. Larry looked like he was near his last breath.*

I chatted with Larry for a while. Then I went out and spoke with the nurses, who said, "Oh, yes, we thought we were going to lose him last night." I spoke with a wonderful resident physician who said, "You know, how long a person lives is up to God. I can tell you the chemistry of what is going on in his lungs, and it's much more complicated than simple pneumonia because of the presence of the cancer and the chemotherapies." I went back and spoke with Larry. I said, "Larry, this looks much more serious." "Yes," he said. "I decided a few days ago that it is my time to go. As I understand it, my choice is to become a patient and be here for the next six to nine months, slowly getting weaker with more complicated tubes. I choose not to do that. I've lived a wonderful life. I've been very successful. I have a great family. I want to die living fully and not as a patient."

I asked Larry if he had discussed his decision with his wife of more than 50 years. "No, she's not ready to hear it yet," he replied. "Larry, this is a pretty big decision," I said. "I think you should share it. Could I have Peg come in, and we'll have a conversation?" He agreed, and Peg joined us. We had a long conversation with many tears. At the end of it, Larry placed a call to a friend, who lent them a house at the beach. Larry then called their children, inviting them and the grandchildren to join him and Peg the next day for a week at the beach house. They left the hospital the next morning and joined their family at the beach. When Larry came home, he wrote letters to all his friends and spoke with them. He died within the next weeks, having lived fully these last days of his life.

What are the implications of Larry's awareness of becoming a patient versus living fully as he comes to the moment of death? What assumptions are challenged by this lived experience of one family – the core phenomena of experience replicated every day in millions of families across the globe?

Assumption Number One: Death is a problem that should be prevented at all costs, no matter how poor the quality of life.

The first assumption that I invite you to question with me is our cultural attitude toward death – that death is an evil to be avoided.

Western medicine is predicated on *death as an evil* to be

avoided at all costs; indeed, a large percentage of our national health-care budget is spent in the last year of life, preventing death at great expense to the individual and to the health-care system and the government, and with great added suffering to the individual and families.[2]

With this assumption, we largely have lost the art of dying. We have lost our understanding of the *signum mortis*. We have a health-care research system predicated on fighting death and with a zero success rate thus far! As one physician put it, "I have never saved a life. I have postponed the moment of death."

The signs of death, *signum mortis,* are a coloring on the face and a presence in the eyes – signs most people recognize when they are in the presence of somebody who is about to die. These signs commonly were understood before they were inadvertently written out of the medical education curriculum with the publication of the Flexner Report in 1910. (Elsewhere, we will talk more about the Flexner Report.) These signs of death routinely are ignored in the modern world. Recently, however, with hospitals requiring individuals to sign papers called "advanced directives" has come an attempt to reawaken knowledge of those signs and of the art of dying (the *Ars Morendi*); we are being reminded of this conversation and of recovering awareness.

Pneumonia used to be known as the elderly person's "friend." Before the age of antibiotics, an elderly person who developed pneumonia would almost surely die from the disease. Now folks in nursing homes who are near death are given antibiotics regularly and thus enabled to suffer longer. An antibiotic is appropriate in some cases, and in others it is not. The ability of physicians and relatives to observe the signs that one is ready to die is critical. That skill is what enabled me to raise the question with Larry.

The choice Larry made had immediate implications for his family. It gave them a chance to have full and rich conversations and to allow the flow of the natural course of his life. We are not talking about euthanasia, and I am not talking about any intervention to hasten death. What I am talking about is allowing the natural course of the disease, rather than setting up a fight.

Larry's decision probably saved the health-care system close to half a million dollars. If you have health-care insurance, Larry and Peg's decision saved you money – all of us would have shared in paying for the additional nine months of Larry's care. Consider the number of days of intensive hospital care. Think of the number of visits to doctors, of x-rays and MRIs, of the medications to slow the cancer and to restore lung function, of rehabilitation after each intensive episode. The cost of this care would have been enormous. Because of Larry's age, those costs would have been borne by Medicare (and thus a portion of it spread to everyone who pays a Medicare tax) and, in Larry's case, by a secondary insurer – probably BlueCross BlueShield (and thus paid by all of those who support that insurer with their premiums).

Most cultures deal with death as part of the cycle of life; and there is some evidence that the significantly lower health-care costs in other developed nations may be due to this difference in cultural attitude: an acceptance of death as part of the cycle of life. In *The Hastings Center Bioethics Briefing Book*, Daniel Callahan documents the evidence that this different attitude toward death lowers costs, and he asks this question: "Should death be seen as the greatest evil that medicine should seek to combat, or would a good quality of life within a finite life span be a better goal?"[3,4]

Our culture's way of dealing with death is in contrast with something my fourth-grade teacher, Sister Jean Marie, spoke every day at the end of school. She would say, "Now, when you go home, be sure you are peaceful and loving with everyone and kiss them goodnight, because we never know who may die during the night, never know that we might not be able to make up for this day in the next day." That wisdom about death was very much a part of my childhood. Death was understood as part of the cycle of life in this neighborhood in New York City; it was reiterated by a fourth-grade teacher in a matter-of-fact way, not as an embarrassment. I often think if a fourth-grade teacher were to say something like that today, she might be dismissed for child abuse.

Story Number Two: Living Well with Disease

I think of Mary, the chief nurse at a major hospital, who had to retire because she had numerous diseases including lupus, high blood pressure, and diabetes. She had amazing physicians who had kept her alive and functional for many years. Finally, she got to the point where she could no longer leave her apartment and where the drug interactions were becoming quite dangerous. Mary was in a fight with her diseases and had enlisted the best of our medical care system in that fight. She was invited to speak to a group of medical students about her experience. About a year before, she had decided to see a nurse healer, Laura, who was also an acupuncturist. What she said to the medical students was, "I'm a miracle. The doctors kept me alive. They were able to contain my diseases so I could live, but I became increasingly less functional. It wasn't until I met Laura that I began to heal; and as you can see, I'm here speaking with you. I'm able to get around. All of my diseases are under control. I'm using much less medication. I am well, including living with all my ailments."

Assumption Number Two: Health is the absence of suffering, symptoms and disease.

One of the major assumptions in dealing with our health-care dilemma is the idea that if we do everything right, we can be "healthy." My mentor, Ivan Illich, taught me the real issue is that life is difficult, that life includes suffering, and that we must learn the art of suffering in order to be well and to live a "healthy life" with our families and communities. Suffering always contains teachings about the art of living. I'm intrigued that Scott Peck's book, *The Road Less Traveled* – one of the bestsellers of the past 30 years – starts with the line, "Life is difficult."

Where did the idea that we could be "healthy" come from? For any of us, hardly a week goes by without some small symptom coming and going; and hardly a year goes by without us having something we could bring to a doctor, an acupuncturist, or someone who might be termed a "health-care professional." And if we look at our evening television news, we see endless ads speaking of symptoms that can be cured by magic bullets. So how did the idea arise that a human could be healthy in the sense of having no suffering, no symptoms, no disease?

Prior to the Industrial Revolution, individuals went to neighbors for help with their symptoms, people who knew herbs and various potions and ways of healing. And there were those in the community who specialized as healers and helpers, as doctors and shamans – but there was not the idea that one could be "healthy" in our modern sense of the word. Traditionally, one understood how to manage one's symptoms and to live well with the difficulties of life.

With the invention of the factory and the paid laborer going to the factory, the idea arose one had to be healthy in order to work. The factory owner had to know who was genuinely ill and unable to work and then attempt to get that person back to work as quickly as possible; and the factory owner had to know who was a malingerer, somebody who was avoiding work. Thus slowly arose the occupation of "company doctor," the health-care provider who helped the employee to get back to work.

The same occurred in China in the 1950s. When Chairman Mao wanted the communes and factories in China to work at full speed, he convened the acupuncture and Chinese medicine leadership, asking them to come up with something now called *A Barefoot Doctor's Manual* – a document designed to maximize the productivity of the workforce, enabling everyone to be active. What happened in the European factory around 1720 occurred in the Chinese commune in 1950: It became a doctrine that we must be "healthy" and that a healthy person is a productive person. So the concept of being healthy is a rather modern invention. Before that time, a human learned the art of "being well in myself," as my English patients would phrase it in 1976.

Being "healthy" has become a certitude and a burden in our culture. Of course, we must look at the definition of being healthy. For our culture it means the absence of any impediments, of suffering, disease, or discomfort. Yet if I ask any audience, everyone agrees that life is filled with pain, suffering, and difficulties. Nortin Hadler, MD, an expert on back pain, says everyone will have back pain two or three times a year. These pains and aches are simply a part of life; if you turn them over to an expert, you move from being a person dealing with life to becoming the disempowered patient of an expert.[5]

It is the modern world that has created the image of the "healthy" life as not having any symptoms. Our option is to redefine health as the quality of life with which we approach our living, our suffering, and our dying (including dying from a serious disease, a process in which we can still be truly healthy). I suggest we abandon the image that if only we eat the right brown rice, take the right vitamins, visit the right healer, do the right exercise, we will have a life without symptoms.

Robert M. Duggan

Story Number Three: Living Fully, No Matter What Life Delivers

Twenty-seven years ago, around 1985, I received a slip of paper regarding a patient that I was about to see; it said I was to see John, a man about age 30, who had been labeled "quadriplegic." I observed myself thinking, "How can I be helpful to someone who is a quadriplegic? Acupuncture can help folks, but what can I possibly do for that?" I went into the room, said hello to John, sat down and asked, "How can I be helpful?" He said, "My body's perfect. There's nothing wrong with my body." I thought, "This is going to be strange." Then John said to me, "My mind is sharp as a tack. I run the computer section of a large bank in Baltimore. After I had my accident at age 15, I trained as a CPA and as a computer expert. My body and my mind are fine. I'm a little off spiritually, though. Do you think acupuncture can help?" I handed John my needles, climbed on the treatment table and said, "John, this is way out of my league."

I knew John for the next 25 years, until he died in 2010. I learned on the first day with him the label he wore had little or nothing to do with John, the person. He had what could be called a pathology, something not functioning in a physiologically normal way. It didn't seem to bother John; he had declared he was fine – and indeed, he was.

A number of years after I first met John (and I would see him regularly, four or five times a year for what he would call a "spiritual clearing"), he retired from the bank, decided to train himself as a high school math teacher, and became a tutor for Sylvan Learning. Then he decided it was time to get married, published personal ads, met a wonderful woman, dated, went off to Florida to get married – all in his wheelchair where he could move only his hands and his head. Never once in all the years I knew John did I hear him complain.

When John died, he was the longest surviving quadriplegic in America. Last year, one of John's friends sent me a message about

40

his death and told me, "John's mother died a few months before he passed. He had promised his mother, back when he had the swimming hole accident, that she would never have to bury him." John lived fully, embracing what life brought him.

Thus we come to the next assumption:

Assumption Number Three: An expert can diagnose us and fix us.

There was no magic fix for John's condition, and yet he lived as if no one had ever told him he was "quadriplegic." He decided not to be limited by the label someone put on him. John did not become his limitations; he lived fully, not expecting a fix and cure.

We all are familiar with the endless TV ads promising cures for diseases – we can get so entranced with them even if we don't know whether or not we have the disease. For a long time I found people in ads for the "purple pill" so attractive that I wanted to take that pill so I could be like them, even though I didn't know what disease I needed to qualify for that pill. I'm also attracted to a vacation in some of the great heart-care hospitals. The ads make them seem like such wonderful places, often encouraging me to come in for tests so I can find out if I qualify. Best of all, they often promise a happy and healthy life "ever after." Of course, these ads tout the importance of consultation with the appropriate expert at every turn along the way, implying I don't know how to live without an expert. The ads also endlessly remind us of the potential side effects of the "purple pill" interventions – death, all sorts of maladies, etc. – so many side effects that we can be desensitized to the serious warnings.

These ads and the responses and attitudes they engender may seem funny; we often joke about such attitudes in our casual conversations. Unfortunately, however, this is serious business. It's about our lives and about how we expend a lot of our national and personal treasure.

In our culture we collapse the distinction between the label of a pathology when it has become established in a person, and the state of that person – their wisdom and ability to deal with life. We have the habit of saying, "I am a cancer survivor," or "I am an arthritic," or "I am an alcoholic," or "I have MS," or "I suffer from Lyme disease." We have begun to identify ourselves with our disease labels. In fact, many individuals find their community by joining groups to learn how best to cope with the disease that they have become. Many doctors and healers will acknowledge that when individuals identify with their labeled disease so closely, they often have no world beyond that label, and thus, if they were healed, they might lose the only community identity they have.

Disease labels are devised by the practitioners of a particular modality with a particular cultural assumption about disease. This labeling enables the practitioners to understand a particular aspect of functioning. "Arthritis," for example, is a very specific, technical description of certain things going on in the biologic body of an individual. It is not a description of the individual. Ten individuals with arthritis will have 10 very different functionings – 10 different lifestyles, 10 different life situations.

A man called me once and asked, "Could acupuncture help with gout?" Yes, I'd seen studies that reported people with gout had been helped, but I said to the man, "I never met gout walking around by itself. It usually comes attached to a very complex individual who has other symptoms and other ailments and also has lots of life issues – from family to money to work to age. So I may be able to help you; and you may be able to manage your gout if you are stronger. You are not your gout."

Another aspect of this conversation is a frequently noted phenomenon that being labeled with a disease can create the disease. I think of what I've been told about two young women: When they were two years old, their mothers brought them to a hospital for the developmentally disabled. The mothers were told that their daughters suffered from cerebral palsy and would spend their lives in wheelchairs. One mother accepted that prognosis. The other mother said to the physicians, "You will never say that again. You will treat my daughter as a normal young woman. We will have her grow up as if there were no diagnosis." Twenty-five years later, that young woman lives with hardly any noticeable disability.

She said that when she was about 17, a doctor slipped, mentioning to her she was a victim of cerebral palsy. She was greatly upset. Although she did have tremors that came when she was tired, she had never thought about herself as diseased – she was functioning fully. She always knew she had abilities different from those of other young people, just as every child is different from others in many ways.

There's an underlying assumption that each pathology or disease factor in the body can be dealt with separately. Alternatively, we can deal with parts of the body in a context of understanding the ecology of the entire body. As we are learning our planet is one environmental unit with everything impacting everything, we also must be very careful the same balancing act occurs for the inner environment – the inner ecology.

This is the case of a woman in her thirties who was sent to me by her internist because she was seeing five specialists: The young woman was struggling with a gynecological problem, low back pain, constricted urination, irritable bowel, and asthma. Her physician began to worry about the interactions of the medications she was taking, and that those interactions were making her worse as they attempted to deal with each of the separate diseases. When I examined the woman from the perspective of an entirely different physiology, the perspective of Chinese medicine, I realized that her lower abdomen was extremely cold to the touch, and her upper abdomen was extremely warm. In other words, the issues of the lower abdomen (bowel, urination, gynecological problem, and low back issues) were coming from the fact that there wasn't enough heat in the lower body, and the asthma was being generated by an excess of heat in the upper body.

When the difference in heat in the upper and lower part of the body was pointed out to the woman, when we pointed out that most of her breathing was very shallow and that she drank a lot of cold fluids, when we taught her how to breathe more deeply and change her food habits, her body responded within a month and then continued on a healing path. At the end, viewing the woman as a whole resulted in an entirely different way of healing; in fact, the core power was within the ability of the woman to shift her daily patterns. In making those shifts, she gained power. She no longer had four or five pathologies – she had symptoms that taught her how to live well.

The way the physician dealt with each condition defined in Western medical terms was appropriate. However, viewing the woman as a whole resulted in an entirely different way of healing.

Story Number Four: Our Choices Create Our Reality

About ten years ago, I was asked to see a very successful businesswoman, one of the top executives of a Fortune 500 company related to the dot-com industry in its heyday. I was especially interested in seeing her because I was told that she had been examined by four of the top complementary doctors in the United States – names we all would know. I thought, "I'll not only get to see the reports about the examinations by mainstream doctors, I'll also get to see these interesting reports from complementary doctors." However, given the circumstances, I doubted I could be of assistance.

The woman came in with symptoms one might categorize as preliminary to multiple sclerosis. It was a severe, debilitating condition, and indeed, something to worry about. I don't recall that she had a specific disease label at that point. MS was hard to diagnose in those days (and MS continues to be hard to define, as are chronic fatigue, lupus, or any of the degenerative diseases).

As we went along the normal course of the examination, her condition did sound very serious. Then I asked her about food. I asked what she had eaten the day before, and she said, "I had a doughnut in the morning. I worked really hard all day and then grabbed a hamburger at McDonald's on the way home, about 11 o'clock at night." I asked her if that was typical, and she said, "Quite often." I then asked what time she got to bed last night. "Well, about 12:30, maybe 1:00." What time did you get up?" "Around 6:00," she said. "How much fluid do you drink?" "I probably don't drink enough water, but I drink a little water and a lot of Coke." "When was the last time you exercised?" She thought for a while and answered, "I went for a walk about three weeks ago." Then I asked, "Did the symptoms ever go away?" Again, she thought for a while and said, "Oh, they completely disappeared for two weeks when I was on vacation in Canada with my friend last year." "So you're telling me you don't get enough food, you drink hardly any fluids except for caffeine, you don't get enough sleep, you don't exercise, and all the symptoms went away when you went on vacation. That's quite fascinating," I said. "I think that perhaps instead of the $100,000 you've spent on all this testing, perhaps a $100,000 vacation might be the beginning of a cure. And then you can begin to look at ways to take care of yourself." We continued in that direction.

Then I read the reports from all the complementary providers. Every single one of them had prescribed for her an herb or other remedy that was, essentially, a stimulant to keep her going. No one had picked up on the fact that she was not taking care of herself; they were more fascinated with figuring out the specialized disease.

Assumption Number Four: Our lifestyle doesn't matter because (we believe) disease functions separately from our activities.

We have an assumption we can keep going, be extremely busy and not have enough sleep, and our body will continue to function in a relatively normal way; and if there is a complication, an expert can prescribe a chemical to make things better. We need to recognize sleep and patterns of sleep in rhythmic order are essential to a good quality of life.

A *New York Times* article on sleep and the marketing tactics of the "sleep-industrial complex" (the article's title) pointed to the value of sleep: "We all might be better off if the industry sold sleep as something to be savored for its own sake . . . ."[6] Similarly, the same can be said about the value of breathing more deeply, making healthy food choices, drinking cleaner water – all the basics of life, the building blocks of wellness.

Our body is always generating minor symptoms. An example: I have five symptoms. My eyes get tired; I might think it's dirty glasses, but eventually I notice that my eyes are tired. If I don't pay attention to the tiredness in my eyes, keep cleaning the glasses and don't get extra rest, then I'll begin to have more frequent urination. If I don't notice that I'm urinating more frequently and am thirstier than usual, the next symptom arises: restless nights and inability to sleep because I'm overly tired. If I don't pay attention to that restlessness, then my left leg will begin to ache. My body is sending me messages about how to behave; it's telling me to respect my leg-ache and get off the leg. However if I again ignore that warning and keep going, my left ankle will speak to me more loudly and become increasingly painful and swollen until I can no longer stand on it. This is a signal that I've been ignoring the wisdom of my body. Over the years I've learned that my body requires 36 hours of total bed rest – and then, at this point, my body will be fine.

A number of years ago, a wonderful, very creative executive

who had suddenly contracted Lyme disease was referred to me. His symptoms were so severe that he had to carry his own portable intravenous antibiotic drip system with him everywhere. The assumption was he had contracted Lyme disease in a place he had frequented for many, many years, and where there were many, many deer and deer ticks. As we explored this assumption, it turned out his symptoms – the effects of a Lyme disease infection – had begun to appear in his body at a time his wife described as the most hectic and pressured of his life. From looking at his situation and hearing many similar anecdotal stories, I suspected (and there's no way to prove it because our research doesn't focus on such possibilities), he probably had been infected for many years, but the infectious agent did not have power over his wellness until he came under this excessive pressure. His story teaches us that we are in a constant balancing act, and must make the assumption that we need to tend our inner wellness to cope with the constant presence of pathogens in the world.

The lesson of the executive is similar to that of children in a first-grade class: Some of them get the flu or a cold, and some do not. How do we explain that? It's clear the answer is more than the presence of "bugs" in the classroom. Otherwise, everyone would get sick.

Conclusion

We operate as a nation from four cultural certitudes which, when examined even superficially, we all understand are nonsensical. In order to have a rational cost-quality-access structure for health care, these assumptions must be examined and new assumptions created. This process requires a major cultural shift in attitudes. Daniel Callahan, in the Hastings Institute book cited above, says, "An astonishing 40 percent of Americans believe that medical technology can always save their lives; many fewer Europeans share this fantasy. The old joke that Americans believe that death is one more disease to be cured is no longer a joke."

For the sake of our grandchildren and to honor our elders, we must act wisely to shift these cultural certitudes.

NOTES

1. Medical anthropologist Claire M. Cassidy, PhD, designed and conducted the first-of-its-kind "Patients' Own Words" research project, which reports what acupuncture users nationwide think of their treatment. Mainly they say it helps them stay well and understand how they are able to control their own symptoms. See the following:
    – Claire Cassidy, "New Research: Patients Vote an Overwhelming 'Yes' for Acupuncture." *Meridians* (Spring 1996).
    – Claire Cassidy, "In the Patients' Own Words: Research Report, Part 2." *Meridians* (Summer 1997).

2. Donald R. Hoover, Stephen Crystal, Rizie Kumar, Usha Sambamoorthi, and Joel C. Cantor, "Medical Expenditures during the Last Year of Life: Findings from the 1992-1998 Medicare Current Beneficiary Survey." *Health Services Research* (December 2002; 37(6): 1625-1642). Also see:
    – Ivan Illich, *Limits to Medicine: Medical Nemesis, The Expropriation of Health* (Marion Boyars Publishers, 2000).
    – Bing Guo, Christa Harstall, "Advance Directives for End-of-Life Care in the Elderly – Effectiveness of Delivery Modes." (Alberta Heritage Foundation for Medical Research, Edmonton, Canada, August 2004).

3. Daniel Callahan, *The Hastings Center Bioethics Briefing Book for Journalists, Policymakers, and Campaigns*, ed. Mary Crowley (Garrison, NY: The Hastings Center, 2008).

4. Daniel Callahan, *The Troubled Dream of Life: In Search of Peaceful Death* (Georgetown University Press, 2000).

5. Nortin M. Hadler, *Stabbed in the Back: Confronting Back Pain in an Overtreated Society* (University of North Carolina Press, 2009).

6. Jon Mooallem, "The sleep-industrial complex." *The New York Times* (November 18, 2007).

What Is a Useful Question?

"The significant problems that we have cannot be solved at the same level of thinking we were at when we created them."
– *Albert Einstein*

THE UNITED STATES of America is the only country in the developed world without efficient and direct access to comprehensive health care for all of its citizens. One president after another has proposed some version of providing increasing access to care; this has been a major political issue for more than 60 years, culminating in the recent Affordable Care Act championed by President Obama. A very complex situation has grown even more confusing, piece-by-piece, over a long period of time.

In the political battle that surrounds this Act, one side says, in essence, that people should fend for themselves and be independent, and that nobody should be required to pay for anybody else's medical care. The other side says access to health care when we are sick is a basic human right, the cost of which must be shared by the entire community. Here we have a profound philosophical divide of balancing the common good and individual rights, a discourse that is far beyond the scope of this essay. However, when I hear such a polarized conversation – such an oppositional way of

speaking, a dialogue that is unsatisfactory to everyone on all sides
– my instinct is that everyone is engaged in the wrong conversation,
that the wrong question is being asked. The larger, undisclosed,
and usually more basic question gets lost behind the smokescreen
of a debate that looks at the future through the issues and problems
of the past. I call this small-minded thinking.

What everyone seems to agree on is that the American health-
care system is in a state of crisis. The intent of this essay is to examine the unexamined, to question the usual, and to look at this
extraordinarily complex issue with a larger mind, to acknowledge
that the usual answers about improved payment systems, hospital
vigilance, security systems and training are not delivering the outcomes – no matter how much we invest.

We must be very thoughtful about where we are and how
we've gotten here, understanding that all that now exists was created by groups of individuals to solve the dilemmas of a previous
age, and that it may not be sufficient to serve the needs of the present moment or as the foundation of future improvement.

The *"If Only"* Answers and Responses

If only we had a single-payer system . . . *If only* we had universal
coverage . . . *If only* the doctors would figure out cures for cancer
and diabetes . . . *If only* practitioners and doctors and nurses spent
more time and took better care of people . . . *If only* the system
worked better . . . *If only* it weren't so complicated . . . *If only*
medicine weren't so expensive . . .

Over the past decades, many efforts have been made to deal
with these "if only" conversations:

- Managed care was supposed to be a solution, to make things
  more efficient and slow down out-of-control costs.

- Congress increased funding for National Institutes of Health (NIH) studies of possible cures; and now, after many years, we discover that many of the cures have their own complications, including side effects and complex drug interactions that may be more dangerous than the original diseases.

- We tried expanded coverage, only to find that more and more tests for patients and more and more drugs carry their own complications.

We don't solve these issues because they're not the right issues to solve, not the right areas of focus – the reason I have refused to do clinical outcomes research because the inquiries are framed in terms of solving the problem of specific diseases. Does acupuncture help asthma? Well, that's an odd question for me to study when my patients with asthma are saying, "Asthma has become my friend that teaches me how to live well." In truth, the right issues are more basic; and it will take great mindfulness to look at the issues differently.

How do we even begin to reduce the complexity of the current system to basic terms, to find the assumptions on which we're basing decisions and get to the questions that will serve? I suggest the following steps for a useful discourse:

1. Let's be thoughtful about what we have accomplished.

2. Let's acknowledge each other for those accomplishments and let go of the past so we can focus on the future.

3. Let's have a conversation for the next steps – a conversation that starts with a blank slate.

4. Then we can decide what the next task is and ask how we are going to accomplish it.

5. Then we can create partnerships for moving forward.

Let's look at these steps to open our way forward in the current situation in American health care, a world where there have been extraordinary accomplishments, extraordinary breakthroughs, and where there is enormous chaos and confusion. I suggest that the terms of the debate are focused on past accomplishments and past problems, and thus unable to focus on steps two and three. Letting go of the past is essential for envisioning and creating a new future.

Being Thoughtful about What We Have Accomplished

We have amazing health care readily available. I tore the quadricipital muscle on my knee. I'm able to go into a hospital one evening, and in the morning, magical people (nurses, anesthesiologists, surgeons) put it back together again. I don't have to know how they did it. After I go home, I get outstanding physical therapy. This is an amazing system, and we can be truly thankful for what we have accomplished in this modern world.

And, despite our magical drugs, technologies and innovations, we have perhaps the worst health system outcomes in the world. Throughout the conversation about the new affordable health care, there has been a constant refrain from political voices: *America has the best health-care system in the world, and we must keep it that way. We can't let changes in the system diminish the fact that we have access to the best health care in the world.* Few people questioned that premise. And it is false. According to reports from the Centers for Disease Control and Prevention, the World Health Organization, the United Nations and other sources, it is clear the United States ranks very low in overall health-care outcomes among the developed nations of the world.[1]

The "best" aspects of our health-care system are available

only to those who can afford to access it. Increasingly, the value of even these aspects is questionable when we see, for example, the evidence for the effectiveness of prostate screening, which shows those with access to the best prostate screening have seen little benefit and perhaps even a danger. Other evidence indicates that the complications from false mammograms and over-testing may not be producing the best life-saving outcomes. This is the work of a number of scholars who are questioning our expenditures on preventive care, and the multiplication of drugs used for various disease factors among those who can afford access to that care.[2.3]

Despite the framing of the debate, every American *does* have *some* access to health care. No one is supposed to be turned away at emergency room doors when in extreme crisis. We already pay for care for everyone; however, we are doing it in the most expensive way possible. I don't know of anyone who opposes universal health care who would stand at the door of a hospital and turn away a mother with a young child who is dying in her arms. Recently, however, we witnessed one state denying coverage for transplants, allowing several individuals to die because they could not cover the costs of a transplant (and in April 2011 reversed that practice). At the same time, we have the federal government authorizing the expenditure of nearly $90,000 per patient for a prostate cancer drug useful for seriously ill individuals, a drug that extends life for only about four months. We have access and we have rationing of care, both of which can be applied with bewildering inefficiency.

We will have formal universal access to health care as of 2014 (unless the law is changed by the Supreme Court or the Congress). These past three years have seen intense debate about "Obamacare" (as labeled by its opponents) and "affordable access care" (as deemed by its proponents). Gallup Poll surveys indicate that Americans are in favor of everyone having access to health care. Yet there is an enormous division about how to provide that care, a division clearly evident in the political battles of the Obama Administration. While the health-care bill passed in 2010, it did so by a narrow margin and was very close to failing, as efforts of President and Mrs. Clinton did in 1993. Further, aspects of the bill are being challenged in the courts. We have passed a universal access bill, as confusing as it is. After many hours of testimony and expert advice from all quarters, as well as the constant attention of the US House of Representatives and the US Senate on this topic for years, we have put in place powerful systems through which everyone will have access to care within the next four- to eight-year period. This has been a conversation about access to care, payment for care, responsibility for payments, taxation, how much it will cost, how to make it more efficient, how to control costs by driving down the costs of care, greater efficiency, the elimination of certain forms of abusive malpractice insurance, etc. This intensive conversation has not addressed whether increased access to a "disease-care" system will actually benefit our society or bankrupt us.

Apparently, the CEO of General Electric, Jeffrey Immelt, thinks it will do the latter – the current system will bankrupt us. In February 2010, he announced to an audience in Cincinnati if current trends continue, " . . . the only employees in Cincinnati will either be working for the hospitals, or lawyers suing the hospitals, or lawyers defending the hospitals." Our entire GDP, he implied, would revolve around health care.[4]

Acknowledging What We Have Done Together

We must acknowledge all that has been accomplished by modern medicine; it is truly miraculous – think of the lives that are prolonged and the suffering that is alleviated. We have an amazing system for acute emergencies – for accidents, broken bones, wounds. In extreme situations, we have helicopters flying to emergency rooms and we have our battlefield medicine. In the realm of acute care, we have accomplished something remarkable that is worth exporting to the rest of the world. However, our accomplishments in acute emergency medicine account for only a tiny portion of the health-care issues and health-care expenditures.

In the past 100 years, humans have created something extraordinary; and in the doing of that great work, we have lost control of the system and perspective of how it operates in relation to our society and our individual lives. There is no one person or group to blame for the present crisis in health care; we are *all* to blame. It's not the doctors who have done this to us. It's not the pharmaceutical companies that have done this to us. Each of us has the desire to be fixed immediately whenever there is discomfort. Each of us has wanted a magic cure. "I want the purple pill advertised on television for whatever disease because the people shown with it are so happy." Each of us wants to live as long as we can. And many of us would like to be able to stay up all night and enjoy television and still get up bright and early in the morning for work. We all are torn between the longing for effortless happiness and our hope to avoid the often hard day-to-day realities of life.

Our desire to do whatever we want to our bodies without consequences is rooted in the larger illusion that we are in charge of our planet, that we are not subject to the laws of nature regarding death and suffering, not subject to the impact of what we eat and to the quality of the air we breathe, that we can mistreat our environment and the planet will recover. These are horribly mistaken assumptions.

In the previous essay, we pointed to four other flawed assumptions that are at the heart of our relationship to our health-care system. I believe the refusal to address those defective assumptions in a serious way are the root of our impasse. We still are attempting to prevent death at all costs, to prevent suffering at all costs, to assume that there is a magical fix for all illnesses, and to pretend our life habits are unrelated to our symptoms and diseases. Those are the underlying assumptions of our health-care system; and in the absence of questioning those assumptions, we are preparing for a constant increase in the percentage of GDP devoted to health care.

Standing back a bit, we can see we have created a massive disease-care system and a relatively tiny disease-prevention system; and in the process we have lost the most basic awareness of how to live well – good food, good play, good exercise, good breathing, good sleep, good friendship, good family life – so very basic that we have lost perspective on how essential they are to good living, and instead have focused on breakdowns and disease. The way we've been dealing with the issue we call "health" is not working and will not work; nor will this path we are on serve our children and grandchildren.

Starting with a Blank Slate

As we've seen, the normal discourse about health care has been one of blaming the other person, blaming the providers who don't listen, blaming the system that is too bureaucratic, blaming the paying system that is too complex, blaming the admissions process. It is a conversation about "if only." It is a conversation that attempts to frame the future solutions around the archaic issues of the past. It is a conversation marred by both deeply philosophical differences and partisan bickering. It is a conversation around a core of false assumptions and questions that lead nowhere.

It is a conversation that has broken down, leaving us . . . where?

Ancient philosophies and the modern organizational development texts (such as *Presence,* by a group of well-known organizational consultants led by Peter Senge and Betty Sue Flowers) point out that in the presence of such breakdown, opposition, and contradiction, one has to go deep into the unknown, into the abyss, letting go of all assumptions. We are at the bottom of a great cycle of life, – the failure of an existing system and a great unknowing about what to do next.[5]

It is only from this frame of mind, without personal or political or financial agendas, and open to all possibility at a moment of enormous new potential and creativity, that "crisis" can truly come to mean "opportunity."

It is only from this frame of mind that we can start to ask new questions: What would we do if we started from zero? What if we had no health-care system? What would we design if the only assumption we started with was the concern for the wellness of our children and grandchildren?

What would we design if we had a blank check? What would we create?

It is with these questions in mind that we are able to and must begin a new conversation.

What can this look like? What new thing can we do together?

Hopeful Possibilities for the Future

There are possibilities for positive change all around us. Most of them are much too simple to be taken seriously in the face of such a massive collapse. Yet we can point to the simple and wonderful things already available to take us in a more sustainable direction. And again, the possibilities arise from asking very different questions.

We are part of the worldwide impact of everybody touching everyone else through our air, soil, foods, lights, patterns. When we realize everything impacts all of us, we might recover the reality that, for the sake of all beings, each of us is fully accountable for living as well as we possibly can, for being our own primary health-care provider, for accepting that our actions do have consequences in the way we breathe and live and in the general quality of our life. *We have to accept the fact that at some point we will die, and we have some control of that passage by the quality of the way we live; and we must awaken to our bodies and acknowledge that part of life is learning to live with pain and stress, learning how to bear, with life's difficulties and moving on.*

This learning can begin at any stage in life; ideally, it begins in early childhood. It means learning how to pay attention to our body – to notice how the food we are eating is creating problems rather than having us feel well; to notice the quality of the air we are breathing, the fluids we are drinking; and to notice when we are lacking in exercise based on the way our body feels. This process of learning involves the delicious reawakening of our senses so we can re-experience how we keep ourselves well. Our bodies are our teachers, and they will guide us to better ways of living.

The payoff for this new possibility is that we might take the $1.2 trillion currently wasted annually by our disease-care focus – to say nothing of the untold trillions wasted by remaining on this course – and redirect a portion of those funds in much more productive ways to promote wellness.[6]

End of a False Conundrum

Think about it in this way: As we have seen, the crux of the breakdown in our current system is that we are paralyzed by cost issues, access issues, and quality issues. A change in any one of these areas changes all the others. For 30-plus years, this puzzle box of cost-access-quality has been known as the iron triangle of the health-care debate and seen as an insoluble dilemma.

I say this is a false dilemma. This conversation assumes increased access to health care is the goal, but we have already examined where that road leads. I propose to intentionally design ways to *reduce* access because over 70 percent of those seeking medical care are in the wrong place. They are being given access to a disease-care system when they need access to a wellness system.

The magic of antibiotics, blood transfusions, and modern surgery distract us from the possibility that the most effective and most cost-efficient health-care system is rooted in the idea of a way of life that maximizes wellness. A lifestyle of wellness will reduce the number of people needing access to the expensive disease-care system. Thus, antibiotics, blood transfusions, modern surgery – powerful and often problematic tools – become the exception rather than the rule, the fallback position rather than the norm.

Achieving this goal might be a matter of awakening base economic instincts. This is already happening. In Senate testimony, Catherine Baase, MD, Global Director of Health Services for Dow Chemical, cited a meta-review of 56 published studies showing an average $5.81 savings for every $1 invested in wellness programs for employees.[7] Think about the lifelong savings that will occur if first-graders are taught yogic breathing and stretching for hyperactivity versus given a sedating drug. This move offers young people a life of breathing (free) versus a lifelong habit of medications (expensive).

It will not be an easy process to shift such basic assumptions. It's akin to learning to drive again if someone switched the position of the gas pedal and the brake pedal. However, this must be done. Full implementation will take many years and many generations.

Already a wellness system is growing in the United States – we just don't yet see it as the alternative world to the disease-care system. We think of spas, massage, yoga classes, organic food, local produce, and exercise programs as luxury items. I say, yes, these are some ways we can prevent some future disease; and their power comes not only from their intrinsic value, but also in their potential to provoke a different way of thinking about life and death, and to engage a strong local, familial support community.

Wellness is not primarily about prevention of disease; it is about living well, slowing down, and being as peaceful as possible in every moment. It is about focusing on what is flourishing, and thus lessening the potential for unnecessary suffering.

I say this challenge to create wellness is much more enlivening with bigger possibilities and greater potential than the current challenge – the challenge of fighting disease and struggling with the erroneous image of the iron triangle that locks in our current health-care system. This wellness challenge brings the excitement of remarkable possibilities of life fully lived in the 21st century.

NOTES

1. See the extensive notes in Essay 4, which fully document this paragraph.

2. Sharon Begley, "Why Almost Everything You Hear About Medicine is Wrong." *Newsweek* (January 23, 2011).

3. Nortin M. Hadler, *The Last Well Person: How to Stay Well Despite the Health-care System* (Mcgill Queens University Press, 2004).

4. Jeffrey Immelt, General Electric Chairman and CEO, is quoted in the *Cincinnati Enquirer*, February 27, 2010, in an article headlined, "GE chief: Let's do health care."

5. Peter M. Senge, C. Otto Scharmer, Joseph Jaworski, Betty Sue Flowers, *Presence: An Exploration of Profound Change in People, Organizations, and Society* (Crown Buisness, 2005).

6. Pricewaterhouse Coopers. "The Price of Excess: Identifying Waste in Healthcare Spending." (www.pwc.com/us/en/healthcare/publications/the-price-of-excess.jhtml).

7. Testimony by Catherine M. Baase, MD, before the Senate Committee on Health, Education, Labor and Pensions on February 23, 2009, is available at www.help.senate.gov.

Again, from a conversation with medical students:

During a recent moment of public discourse about the possibility of a worldwide pandemic, I was challenged by a group of medical students as to what natural medicine could offer that would be as effective as a vaccine (which would take many months to develop). I suggested that perhaps the most effective emergency intervention would be to close down the electric grid for nine hours every night so everyone would get more sleep and thus have their immune system strengthened and their stress levels reduced, both of which build effective levels of disease resistance. The students clearly were thrown off by the emphasis on wellness rather than on the usual image of starting a battle with disease. This was certainly a different answer to a different question from a different perspective.

The Health-care Monopoly

"If these fundamental principles can be made clear . . . to those who govern the colleges and the universities, we may confidently expect that the next ten years will see a very much smaller number of medical schools in this country, but a greatly increased efficiency in medical education, and that during the same period medical education will become rightly articulated with, and rightly related to, the general educational system of the whole country."[1]
– Abraham Flexner, 1910

WHEN WE SPEAK of and debate "health care" or "medicine" or "modern medicine," most of us are unaware that we are actually referring to only one of the many systems of medicine available to us. "Modern medicine" is a monopoly created over the past 100 years. In the eighteenth century and into the early nineteen hundreds when homeopathic physicians were prominent, the word for the burgeoning system of medicine that we're familiar with today was "allopathy." Treating disease allopathically was to coerce the body into doing something it would not normally do by introducing a chemical in order to counteract the symptoms. This allopathic approach is very powerful and rooted philosophically in a very different perspective of the human body than homeopathy, a system that considers the person as a whole and enhances the individual's natural responses to neutralize the effects of pathogens. And these are only two of many world-class systems of medicine.

Homeopathy exists today in the shadow of the allopathic monopoly, but it was once a popular and broadly respected form of American medicine. At one time many members of the US Congress were homeopaths; and indeed the homeopathic pharmacopoeia was protected by Congress and is still protected under American law. Yet most contemporary Americans are unaware of this alternative to our disease-care system.

In addition to allopathic medicine and homeopathy there are many other great traditions of medicine, including the extraordinary physiology and medical delivery system of Chinese Medicine, recognized by a Texas court judge in a landmark 1980 decision on the freedom of health-care choice:

> *Acupuncture has been practiced for 2000 to 5000 years. It is no more experimental as a mode of medical treatment than is the Chinese language as a mode of communication. What is experimental is not acupuncture, but Westerners' understanding of it and their ability to utilize it properly.*

> *U.S. District Court for the Southern District of Texas*
> *Andrew vs. Ballard, 498 F Supp. 1038*
> *(S.D. Tex. 1980)*

Among the many other medical systems are Ayurvedic medicine, developed by the great cultures of India, and Hippocratic medicine, an older Western system that preceded allopathy. (Hippocratic medicine, rooted in Greece and traditions from Persia and the Middle East, is a humoral medicine that dominated Europe into the 1700s and remained popular in some circles through the 1900s.)

In our country, committed to capitalism, we are conditioned to reject the practice of monopoly on the corporate level; and our system of government and academic freedoms ensure we are free to explore a variety of ideas and inquiries, thus prohibiting monopolies of thought. *And yet, the way we think about medicine is a de facto monopoly.* True, there is a lively competition within our medical system among hospitals, doctors, pharmaceutical companies, and surgeries; however, seeing so much competition for the most exciting pill or hospital, we may not recognize all this competition exists within a particular allopathic monopolistic perspective. The great diversity of care that existed in the nineteenth century has disappeared. The homeopathic hospitals, once prevalent, have disappeared. For example, the allopathic Hahnemann Hospital in Philadelphia originally opened as a homeopathic hospital named for the founder of homeopathy. Osteopathic schools merged into being essentially allopathic medical schools. Chiropractors had to fight the AMA all the way to the Supreme Court in order to gain a relatively equal footing with the allopathic system; many years later, however, they still are largely overshadowed by that system.

The allopathic monopoly on our thinking and pocketbooks is similar to the kind of monopoly that Ma Bell (AT&T) exerted before anyone thought of alternative forms of electronic communication: When MCI first offered a different kind of phone service, they challenged the all-consuming monopoly of AT&T and eventually paved the way for the innovations in communication that have changed the world. We take this diversity for granted today. Similarly, consider fossil fuels, another virtual monopoly on our highways and power grid since their widespread adoption in the 1800s. Today, we understand the use of such resources is unsustainable, and we are branching out to find effective alternatives that will keep us going.

We are in a similar situation in health care. The existing conversation is so pervasive we can hardly imagine it is only one of many possible conversations about health, only one of many possible systems of care – just as we could not have realistically imagined solar power or mobile phones 40 years ago.

Medicine was standardized from 1910 up to the modern times. I would like to believe what occurred was inadvertent, that the standardization of the ways of examining outcomes and effectiveness of medicine (a very reasonable and laudable goal) resulted from the unwitting limitations of the systems to which standardization was applied. The result of this move was that those who were not practicing standardized allopathic medicine – even those who were highly effective and attained better outcomes with practices that were not allopathic – were proclaimed a charlatan, a snake oil salesman, a quack. In the desire for quality, entire systems were dismissed. Quality medicine became synonymous with allopathic medicine. And in this monopoly, we all suffer.

How This Happened

When I was a young boy growing up in the Washington Heights area of Upper Manhattan, families had wisdom about how to care for various illnesses. I clearly remember my father sweating me through pneumonia when I was seven years old. There were no antibiotics; he piled on the blankets and forced me to drink hot fluids in an attempt to induce the sweating that would break the fever. He did this himself, probably with the advice of the neighbors and using traditions/methods passed down. We rarely saw a doctor or went to the hospital; and if we did have to enter the medical system, it was a very scary thing – it was admitting that someone was going to die. Instead, the community took care of each other on a daily basis.

Throughout history, there have always been members of the

community who knew various remedies and ways of helping each other get well. Some had more expertise than others; every tribe had a shaman, a healer, a wise person who knew the herbs. And medicine was also a social phenomenon, with an understanding among the populace about what practices would support or inhibit well-being – an understanding that began to fade with the rise of industrialization.

It was industrialization that took the responsibility for wellness away from the communities and put it in the hands of a privileged class; and it was industrialization that began the custom of placing a financial value on an individual's health – if not for the person himself, then for his employer. Ivan Illich points to the first formal health-care worker as the person in the factory in the 1700s assigned the job of deciding which worker could miss a day's labor to recover from an illness, and which person had to get out of bed and go to work – a system that cut down on malingering and increased industrial production. This led to the idea of inducing those who were ill to get back to work quickly to keep to a minimum the expense of replacing and training laborers. An almost identical phenomenon occurred in the People's Republic of China in the 1950s when Mao wanted the communes to be more productive. He ordered the development of the barefoot doctor training programs that would carry basic Chinese medicine – acupuncture and herbs – into the communes, thereby maximizing efficiency by reducing the loss of productive work time.

In the late 1800s there were many different systems of healing, some effective and some not. In England, *caveat emptor* prevailed: consumer beware. In that capitalist system it was the consumer's responsibility to vet credentials and reputations of the various kinds of practitioners available to him. A more modern, scientific approach gained supremacy in Germany, a tradition brought to Harvard and the Johns Hopkins University in the United States.

William Osler, who is memorialized at Johns Hopkins as the father of modern medicine, was a product of his time when it was still possible to blend science with the art of shamanism. Osler is credited with the first use of diagnostic instruments such as the microscope as a part of the diagnostic process, and that is largely what he is remembered for today. He also said, quoting Hippocrates, that the physician should "treat the patient that has the disease, not the disease that has the patient." He became so frustrated by the increasing regimentation at Johns Hopkins that he left to complete his years as a professor of medicine at Oxford University in England. There he treated the son of a friend, an 11-year-old boy refusing to eat, on the verge of death. Osler showed up in full academic regalia every day for weeks to feed the young man, who eventually recovered. The regular appearance of this strange man in the funny garments seemed to be the deciding factor, the intervention that healed. Science or shamanism? Wisdom or snake oil? Healing or modern medicine?

William Osler lived at the end of one era and before the allopathic monopoly was established.

The Flexner Report

In 1910, Professor Abraham Flexner, acting under the aegis of the Carnegie Foundation, produced a book-length study on medical education in the United States and Canada. This report "called on American medical schools to enact higher admission and graduation standards, and to adhere strictly to the protocols of mainstream science in their teaching and research." At that time, "many American medical schools fell short of the standards advocated in the Report, and subsequent to its publication, nearly half of such schools merged or were closed outright. The Report also concluded that there were too many medical schools in the USA, and that too many doctors were being trained." Through this report, Flexner instigated the birth of modern medical education with new standards for training and treatment.[1,2]

The Flexner Report was developed and written in a world of health care that had great diversity. Backed by wealth and the voices of powerful individuals, this report operated from a very particular philosophic stance about science and effectiveness, about what was right and what was wrong. Highly influenced by reductionist attitudes toward science, it focused on how medicine was effective and "Do we understand the mechanisms?" I'm not sure that those who funded the report or Flexner himself reflected on the philosophical issues involved. Modern peer-reviewed articles question Flexner's qualifications to do this report and also question the motives behind the funding of the report; but that discussion would be a distraction. Our reality is that the report took a powerful stance favoring an allopathic approach to medicine – an approach focusing on "fixing" symptoms, an approach assuming that science could solve all the problems.

Whether intentional or inadvertent, the Flexner Report had a dramatically adverse effect on the healing arts that are rooted in the understanding of the human organism's relationship to nature – approaches focusing on natural, low-tech interventions as distinct from high-tech, biochemical interventions. Clearly, the focus on allopathic and high-tech intervention has brought great benefits. However, these great benefits have come at the cost of losing other streams of healing based on great wisdom traditions.

Standard does not necessarily mean *effective*. I remember when my father almost died from an allergic reaction to the standard dose of penicillin he received shortly after World War II, a time when negative reactions to these medicines were already being documented. But the optimistic mood of the 1950s and 60s assumed we humans would create a better world through chemistry, that the new miracle medicines would, along with advances in transportation and food processing, create a utopian future. There was no turning back "progress."

The increasing use of the medical system and of higher-cost medicines eventually required increased insurance coverage for health care. I remember when this began to happen. My father was a union laborer; and despite our previous history of relying on family and neighbors for cures, we began to see doctors more and more often as the unions negotiated for coverage. The late 1960s brought America's first modern battle over universal coverage for health care and the compromise of Medicare and Medicaid.

Progress in medicine – the search for the perfect delivery system for the perfect medicine to prevent all suffering, disease, and death – became even more expensive in the 1980s with the advent of spiraling double-digit inflation in health care. The HMO idea, the original concept of which was preventive wellness, exploded on the scene as a way of controlling costs by eliminating all "inefficiency" from the system. This is another way of referring to increased standardization of care, eliminating the variables of patient choice of their provider, and micromanaging the decision-making process of physicians. (The genesis of such control as a major factor occurred in 1987 at the Allied Signal Corporation. When faced with a 15 percent increase in health-care costs, the chief executive responded with "Zero!" After many negotiations, the response was: "We can do zero, but only if we can control exactly how the care is delivered to everyone." The CEO's personal doctor was replaced with a standard company doctor.)

It was also in the 1980s that I personally witnessed another aspect of this standardization process. As an acupuncturist I had spent the previous decade helping to carve out a place for our alternative to mainstream allopathic care. Parts of the modern medical system realized the threat we posed to their monopoly on medical thinking; they responded by declaring acupuncturists to be surgeons under their jurisdiction because we pierced the skin with steel needles.

In many places it was illegal to practice acupuncture; in places where it was legal, it was declared experimental and thus practiced under conditions that restricted its availability to the public. In order to please the state legislators who wanted to regulate acupuncturists, those of us who were practicing acupuncture had to devise a standardized system of testing. We employed the Professional Examination Service on Riverside Drive in New York City, which developed standardized tests for most professions in the United States.

As we sat at the table discussing those tests, we realized there was great diversity of practice and thought within Chinese medicine, that most of it was a living practice of varied traditions focused on patient outcomes, and that many great traditions from Korea, Japan, China, and Vietnam would be lost if we picked only certain texts on which graduates would be examined – and yet, that was exactly what we had to do to stay out of jail. We didn't have the resources to challenge the existing monopoly and help restore a great panoply of healing diversity, making it available to the American public.

Instead, the narrow focus of standardization, whittling down the possibilities, won the day once again. For the sake of credibility and the appearance of quality, an extraordinary diversity of methods of care (and indeed, less invasive methods of care) essentially were made to disappear – much like what happened when chiropractic and osteopathic medicine were forced into mimicking the diagnostic, disease-focused approach of allopathy. In the words of William Osler, they had begun treating "the disease that has the patient" rather than "the patient who has a disease." While it is important to control for fraud and quackery by establishing performance criteria, it appears that with the application of standardized testing in the USA, much of Chinese medicine will be standardized, wiping out 4,000 years of enrichment through diversity.

The Advent of Universal Health Care

The 1990s brought us more combat over universal health care, this time initiated by then-President Clinton and the First Lady, Hillary. Their attempt, a signature campaign promise, triggered fierce turf battles among the politicians, the medical industry, the hospital industry, the pharmaceutical industry and the consumer industry, which resulted in a collapse of that conversation but left in place the basic dilemma of what is considered the unbreakable iron triangle of cost-quality-access: *If you increase access, either the cost goes up or the quality goes down. If you increase quality, the costs go up but access may go down. If you attempt to control costs, both quality and access go down. This has been the crux of the debate for proponents of universal health coverage* – if the huge numbers of uninsured are covered, it can only be done by a deterioration of quality and access. (As strategizing occurs within the bounds of the allopathic medical monopoly, however, the greater affordability of an alternative medical or wellness system is yet to be considered.)

Now that legislation has been passed providing universal access – a long-time political issue – we may be ready to deal with the even more dramatic problem of the costs of such access and of the quality of care. Attention is moving in that direction. Deval Patrick, the Governor of Massachusetts where they have had universal care since 2006, was quoted as saying, "We must now take on the cost issue."[3,4] Recently I was with a group of health-care executives where the head medical officer reported several instances in which they had been so successful in keeping patients out of the hospital through preventive care and wellness care that the hospitals were in danger of collapsing for lack of business. We are beginning to head in the direction of promoting wellness, simply because it will become an economic necessity.

The Past Fifty Years

For the past fifty years there's been the thought that we can solve the health-care dilemma if only we made the allopathic monopoly more perfect, if we gave it better databases, better technology, more efficiency, and of course, more money. In other words, more standardization and less diversity. But these are solutions based on the existing conversations, which are guaranteed to give us more of the same outcomes. They are solutions keeping us on the same road to health-care debacle and financial ruin – on the same road in a disintegrating vehicle that continues to accelerate.

In my life I've witnessed the transformation of medicine in this country from what was essentially a community-based, common-sense wellness paradigm (even in New York City) to the current highly managed, highly mechanical, rigidly standardized, insanely expensive system we have today. The irony is, with all of this so-called progress, the outcomes are not very different than they were 70 years ago – and possibly they are much worse, as we shall explore in another essay. Not only do we have to live with many of the same symptoms as we did then (as well as many new ones unique to our modern world), we have to live with the side effects and unforeseen interactions of the modern interventions – and all of this in a bloated system that treats us like cogs in a machine and bankrupts us in the process.

I often wonder what the world would be like if there had been no Flexner Report in 1910. I like to think that we would have a thriving competition among allopathic hospitals, homeopathic hospitals, osteopathic hospitals, and chiropractic centers, along with forms of health care such as Chinese medicine, Ayurvedic medicine, and forms of ancient Hippocratic medicine. It is no accident that even though the Rockefeller family was a part of the group that sponsored and supported the Flexner Report and the ensuing standardization of health care, I'm told that up until the late 1960s they kept a clinic in New York City where a great diversity of health-care options were available to family members, including alternatives to the standardized allopathic medicine. It is to Laurance Rockefeller's credit that in the later years of his life he became one of the great supporters of renewed diversity in medicine.

Without the Flexner Report and without this massive intervention from 1910 through 1920, we likely would live in a world with great diversity of health care. Conversations about health care would focus on patient outcomes and life benefit rather than on double-blind studies and cause. Competition among styles and cultures of health care would have been the natural way to restrain costs and to keep the public focused on what best served one's health, rather than on what met the image of a particular set of philosophical assumptions. By recognizing and acknowledging we have developed a monopoly, we now have some power to begin to change the conversation.

NOTES

1. Abraham Flexner, "Medical Education in the United States and Canada. A Report to the Carnegie Foundation for the Advancement of Teaching." Bulletin Number 4, 1910 (D. B. Updike, The Merrymount Press, Boston, reproduced in 1960 and 1972).

2. Mark D. Hiatt, MD, "Around the continent in 180 days: The controversial journey of Abraham Flexner." *The Pharos* (Winter 1999). Available through www.alphaomegaalpha.org/the_pharos.

3. "Health Care in Massachusetts Turns to Cost Control." Interview on NPR, February 14, 2012. Available at www.npr.org/2012/02/14/146848077/health-care-in-massachusetts-turns-to-cost-control.

4. "Deval Patrick on Health Care." Excerpts from Massachusetts 2012 State of the State Address, January 23, 2012. Available at www.ontheissues.org/governor/Deval_Patrick_Health_Care.htm.

A Disaster *for* America

Life expectancy in the United States is ranked 50th in the world,
below most developed nations and some developing nations.[1]
– CIA World Factbook

". . . do no harm."
– Hippocrates

OUR NATION IS in grave danger from the current design of our health-care system. The cost is driving us toward bankruptcy, even while 50 million of us have no access to care without becoming seriously ill. For those of us who do get care, the quality of what we receive ranks very low among all nations, not just among developed nations. The president of a small American hospital was quoted recently as saying, "How is it possible that a rural hospital in India is able to have better outcomes for their patients at 20 percent of the cost?"

It is not the purpose of these essays to document in minute detail a problem that is widely reported. Numerous other resources describe the serious nature of our national crisis. Perhaps the most powerful of these is an article by Ezekiel Emanuel as far back as the May 2007 issue of the *Journal of the American Medical*

Association (JAMA). Here we have one of the most prestigious mainstream medical journals in the United States, overseen by the most powerful medical lobby in the United States, publishing an editorial article by an appointee of the National Institutes of Health, a bioethicist who simultaneously earned an MD and PhD at Harvard, taught at Harvard Medical School, served as Special Advisor for Health Policy to the Office of Management and Budget, and now heads the Department of Medical Ethics and Health Policy at the University of Pennsylvania. In the JAMA article titled "What Cannot Be Said on Television About Health Care," Emanuel speaks directly to politicians and policymakers:

> *"It used to be an accepted trope for U.S. politicians to puff up their chests and pronounce that the United States had the best health care system in the world. . . .*
>
> *"Politicians could say such things because Americans believed them. Even if people somehow knew there were problems, there was a sense that the United States had the best – that those who were rich and could afford anything or were admitted to one of America's great teaching hospitals were getting the best health care available anywhere in the world.*
>
> *"This is no longer true. Many no longer believe the United States has the best health care system in the world."*[2]

By any measure we do have the most expensive system. In 2005 health care in the USA cost each individual more than $6,000 for a total in excess of 16 percent of our gross domestic product (GDP).[3] By 2011 that cost had risen to over $8,000 per person. In the 2005 data, our nearest rival, Switzerland, spent $4,077 per person per year, or 11.5 percent of its GDP; and Germany spent only $3,043 (10.6 percent of GDP).[4] This disparity in cost among highly developed economies should engender serious concern. Americans increasingly are aware that this rate of expenditure of our national treasure is not producing a commensurate return on investment.

Americans are reading in their press that the care they receive is not of the highest quality. The National Institute of Medicine report, *To Err Is Human,* states that 100,000 Americans die each year from medication errors in the hospital. For a wide spectrum of the public, that statistic was emblematic of the overall quality of our health care.[5]

With all our high-tech medical miracles, the United States fails its citizens on the three most basic outcome measures: quality, access, and cost – the three sides of our iron triangle of health-care policy. Here is a very brief recounting of the evidence of systemic failure:

Quality

1. The World Health Report 2000, *Health Systems: Improving Performance,* ranked the US health-care system 37th in the world.[6] It is clear from recent political debates our situation is worse than in 2000.

2. Preventable medical mistakes and infections are responsible for about 200,000 deaths in the US each year according to an investigation by the Hearst media corporation.[7]

3. According to the 2011 *CIA World Factbook,* the United States ranks 176th in the world in infant survival.[8]

4. In 2010, the United States ranked 42nd in the world for its under-five mortality rate, lower than most of Europe, including countries with far fewer resources such as Estonia, Croatia, and Hungary.[9]

5. Life expectancy in the United States is ranked 50th in the world, below most developed nations and some developing nations.[8]

6. Nearly half of all Americans now use prescription drugs on a regular basis, according to a CDC report. Nearly a third of Americans use two or more drugs, and more than one in ten regularly use five or more prescription drugs. The report also revealed one in five children regularly are given prescription drugs, and nine out of ten seniors are on drugs.[10] A prescription drug can be powerful and potentially dangerous. We are well aware of the difficulties in protecting ourselves from drug interactions; we hear endless notices about side effects and the potential dangers of using such drugs. Yet many consider drugs as miraculous, despite well-documented complications and dangers, not to mention the high cost of these medications.[11] A survey of Minnesota residents 65 and over found that the average number of prescription drugs taken daily by seniors is 2.9. The study, reflective of trends throughout the US, indicated that more than one in five seniors take five or more different prescription drugs every day.[12]

Access

1. A record 50.7 million residents (which includes 9.9 million non-citizens), or 16.7 percent of the population, were uninsured in 2009 according to the Census Bureau.[13] A more recent report indicates a decline in that number by one million individuals due to provisions of the 2010 Health Reform Act that enable young adults to remain longer on family policies.[14]

2. The USA is the only wealthy, industrialized nation that does not ensure that all citizens have coverage (i.e., some kind of

private or public health insurance), according to a report prepared by the National Institute of Medicine. The 2004 report observed that "lack of health insurance causes roughly 18,000 unnecessary deaths every year in the United States."[15] A 2009 Harvard study estimated nearly 45,000 annual deaths are associated with lack of health insurance.[16] Even though people eventually will get access to the emergency room, that access is often too late, resulting in complications and deaths. Delayed access is almost a guarantee of poor quality outcomes including unnecessary loss of life.

Cost

1. In 2009 the United States federal, state and local governments, corporations and individuals together spent $2.5 trillion, $8,047 per person, on health care. This amount represented 17.3 percent of the GDP, up from 16.2 percent in 2008.[17] The nearest country in percent of GDP is Sweden at about 11 percent of GDP.[18]

2. The Congressional Budget Office projects that, in the absence of changes in federal law, total spending on health care would rise from 16 percent of GDP in 2007 to 25 percent in 2025, 37 percent in 2050, and 49 percent in 2082.[18]

3. Many would blame General Motors' recent collapse and need for restructuring on the outsize cost of health-care benefits for its current and retired employees. Similar costs are not borne by their major competitors – Toyota, Hyundai or Volkswagen – companies based in countries that provide health care to all citizens. Heath care is one of the most expensive overheads paid by US employers, and a hindrance to global competitiveness.

4. Approximately 25 percent of all Medicare expenditures go to providing care in the last year of life, approximately $39,000 per individual. Approximately 63 percent of all elderly spend time in the hospital in the last months of life.[20] These expenditures provide much valuable and beneficial care; however, it is widely recognized that a significant portion is spent prolonging unnecessary suffering versus enabling an individual to die a reasonable and dignified death.

5. "Treatment for people with chronic diseases and conditions accounts for about 75 percent of the [dollars] spent annually on medical care in the US. According to a 2007 report from Milken Institute on the economic burden of chronic disease, even modest reductions in preventable risk factors could lead to 40 million fewer cases of illness and to savings of more than $1 trillion by 2023."[21] Remember these are annual savings and are based on "modest reductions in preventable risk factors." Imagine the savings by tending these diseases (now often referred to as non-communicable diseases) not as a disease, but rather as an issue of lifestyle choice, which can be tended by changes in lifestyle.[22]

Failure on All Sides of the Triangle

We are failing as a nation in all aspects of the triangle. Many wonderful individuals have devoted themselves to resolving this dilemma. I think of the recent administrator of the Centers for Medicare & Medicaid Services (CMS), Donald Berwick, MD. Dr. Berwick was given a recess appointment by President Obama, but the US Senate did not vote to confirm his appointment on a permanent basis. The CMS, which controls close to 50 percent of our national healthcare expenditures, has not had a permanent full-time administrator since 2006 – a sign of the national gridlock on health-care policy.

Thus as a nation we are failing on quality, cost, and access. An editorial headlined "The High Cost of Health Care" in the *New York Times,* November 25, 2007, states: "It is the worst long-term fiscal crisis faced in the nation, and it demands a solution, but finding one will not be easy or palatable." The editorial ends by observing, "By now it should be clear that there is no silver bullet to restrain soaring health care costs. A wide range of contributing factors need to be tackled simultaneously . . . ." This reality is a serious danger to our entire national economy.

For those who want to explore this topic further, I recommend books by Shannon Brownlee and Nortin Hadler, MD:

- Shannon Brownlee. *Overtreated: Why Too Much Medicine Is Making Us Sicker and Poorer* [23]

Three books by Nortin Hadler:

- *The Last Well Person: How to Stay Well Despite the Health-Care System* [24]

- *Worried Sick: A Prescription for Health in an Overtreated America* [25]

- *Stabbed in the Back: Confronting Back Pain in an Overtreated Society* [26]

Dear reader, if at this point you do not agree we are in serious trouble, please stop reading. If you agree that the serious nature of our national health-care problem requires asking new questions in new ways, then I invite you to explore the following essays with an open and curious mind. I believe they offer a path filled with creative and practical possibilities.

NOTES

1. *CIA World Factbook.* Available at www.cia.gov/library/publications/the-world-factbook.

2. Ezekiel Emanuel, "What Cannot Be Said on Television About Health Care" (*Journal of the American Medical Association,* May 15, 2007, Vol 297, No. 19).

3. Catlin A, Cowan C, Heffler S, Washington B; National Health Expenditures Accounts Team. "National health spending in 2005: The slowdown continues." Available at content.healthaffairs.org/content/26/1/142.full.

4. Organisation for Economic Co-operation and Development. *OECD Health Data 2006: Statistics and Indicators for 30 Countries.* See www.oecd.org.

5. Committee on Quality of Health Care in America, Institute of Medicine, *To Err Is Human: Building a Safer Health System* (National Academies Press, 2000).

6. The World Health Report 2000. Available at www.who.int/whr/2000/en/.

7. "Hearst national investigation finds Americans are continuing to die in staggering numbers from preventable medical injuries," August 9, 2009 report. Available at www.hearst.com/press-room.

8. *CIA World Factbook.* Available at www.cia.gov/library/publications/the-world-factbook.

9. Report prepared by the Institute for Health Metrics and Evaluation. Available at www.healthmetricsandevaluation.org/news-events/news-release/unexpected-decline-newborn-mortality-drives-child-deaths-below-8-million.

10. US DHHS Centers for Disease Control, National Center for Health Statistics, *NCHS Data Brief,* No. 42, (September 2010, p1).

11. Mike Adams, "Americans drowning in prescription drugs." Available at www.naturalnews.com/029664_prescription_drugs_Americans.html.

12. "How are older Minnesotans using prescription drugs?" 2001 survey available on the Minnesota Board on Aging website, www.mnaging.org.

13. Avery Johnson. "Recession Swells Number of Uninsured to 50.7 Million." *The Wall Street Journal* (September 17, 2010, p.A4).

14. "One Million Young Adults Gain Health Insurance in 2011 Because of the Affordable Care Act." Brief issued by the US Department of Health & Human Services, September 2011. Available at aspe.hhs.gov/health/reports/2011/DependentCoverage/ib.shtml.

15. "Insuring America's Health: Principles and Recommendations," 2004 report from the Institute of Medicine of the National Academies. Available at www.iom.edu/Reports.aspx.

16. David Cecere, "New study finds 45,000 deaths annually linked to lack of health coverage." (Summary of a study conducted by the Harvard Medical School and the Cambridge Health Alliance). Available at news.harvard.edu/gazette/story/2009/09.

17. "National Health Expenditures 2009 Highlights." Available at www.cms.gov/nationalhealthexpenddata/downloads/highlights.pdf.

18. Hans Maarse, "Testing Market Practices." Available on The Hastings Center website, healthcarecostmonitor.thehastingscenter.org/hansmaarse/testing-market-practices.

19. "The Long-Term Outlook for Health Care Spending." Study issued by the Congressional Budget Office. Available at www.cbo.gov/ftpdocs/87xx/doc8758/maintext.3.1.shtml.

20. Data from the Centers for Medicare and Medicaid Services, published by Health Research and Educational Trust in a research brief by Gerald Riley and James Lubitz, "Long-term trends in Medicare payments in the last year of life." *Health Services Research* (April 2010, Volume 45, No. 2). Available at www.thefreelibrary.com.

21. Quote from "Creating a Culture of Healthy Living," a document available at www.cdc.gov/HealthyCommunitiesProgram.

22. See the following resources for data, analyses, and strategies regarding health care:

– Milken Institute, "An Unhealthy America: the Economic Burden of Chronic disease. Charting a New Course to Save Lives and Increase Productivity and Economic Growth." Executive Summary and Research Findings, October 2007. Available at http://www.milkeninstitute.org/healthreform/pdf/AnUnhealthyAmericaExecSumm.pdf.
– American Medical Association, "Getting the most for our health care dollars. Strategies to address rising health care costs." A series of publications by the AMA available at www.ama-assn.org/ama/pub/about-ama/strategic-issues/health-care-costs.page.
– Partnership for Solutions, Johns Hopkins University, "Chronic Conditions: Making the Case for Ongoing Care." Available at www.partnershipforsolutions.org/DMS/files/chronicbook2004.pdf.
– National Center for Chronic Disease Prevention and Health Promotion, "Creating a Culture of Health Living." Available at www.cdc.gov/HealthyCommunitiesProgram.

23. Shannon Brownlee, *Overtreated: Why Too Much Medicine is Making Us Sicker and Poorer* (Bloomsbury Press, 2008).

24. Nortin M. Hadler. *The Last Well Person: How to Stay Well Despite the Health-care System* (McGill-Queens University Press, 2004).

25. Nortin M. Hadler. *Worried Sick: A Prescription for Health in an Overtreated America* (University of North Carolina Press, 2008).

26. Nortin M. Hadler. *Stabbed in the Back: Confronting Back Pain in an Overtreated Society* (University of North Carolina Press, 2009).

Note that NIH budget information is available on the National Institutes of Health website at www.nih.gov/about/budget.htm.

Language and Ideas *that* Do Not Serve

"Here's a bold prediction for the new year. By 2020, the American health insurance industry will be extinct. . . . Already, most insurance companies barely function as insurers. . . . All that insurance companies do is process billing claims."[1]
– Ezekiel Emanuel and Jeffrey Liebman, from "The End of Health Insurance Companies"

RECENTLY I HAD the privilege of spending an hour and a half with a young man in his mid-twenties who was about to get married. His fiancée insisted he learn about acupuncture and experience treatment in that modality. He was resistant, but out of his love for her – and out of curiosity aroused by her conviction he should experience acupuncture – he came. I found the conversation quite helpful for my learning and hopeful for him. I observed this young man, George, was trapped in a series of modern assumptions that may be very destructive to his ability to live well, to live fully in his relationships, to serve his future children, and to live a long life gracefully into old age.

George said, "I'm very healthy. I'm very active. I have no

disease, no illness. I work out. I exercise to make sure that I don't get ill. My life is full and wonderful, so I don't really understand why I'm here. I prefer to stay away from doctors. I watch out for myself, and my life is good." As I listened to these words I thought of Nortin Hadler and his book, *The Last Well Person,* in which he asserts that one of the most dangerous things you can do before age 85 is to let an expert diagnose you – a doctor, an acupuncturist, an herbalist, or anyone who attempts to tell you how you are. In essence, George, in his youthful wisdom, seemed to be aware of what Dr. Hadler points to: We have an inner knowing of how to be well.[2]

Yet as I spent time with George, I began to realize my young friend does not have a series of observational life skills that I believe Dr. Hadler assumes are available. George said to me, "I have no illness. I have no symptoms. I'm just fine." And I said to him, "I've never met someone with no symptoms." George seemed to be unaware of his body. Over the years I've found that as I speak with people, they become aware they have many preclinical symptoms they have ignored. Modern individuals have learned to ignore their body unless it screams very loudly for serious attention.

Over the course of our conversation, we discovered there were many symptoms that appeared when George did not get a certain amount of rest, and he often ignored those symptoms. We also learned George sometimes made changes in the kind of food and amounts of food he ate, and he didn't know why this was happening. Further, he repeatedly observed situations where "my heart was racing – my heart jumped out of my chest," a set of symptoms that show up when he is very excited and busy, and that also arise when he is angry and frustrated. As I questioned, he began to realize frustration and anger were emotions he didn't know how to control, so they often went unexpressed or were expressed automatically in the form of sensations in his chest. He was concerned about the sensations but had never observed the link to his emotions.

Further discussion revealed that although he was without a disease label, he was not "healthy." In fact, it became clear he was pushing what he called his "machine-like body" toward a disease that eventually would make him a fit subject for the medical system. Far from living up to his masquerade of enduring good health, he had been ignoring serious symptoms for years because he was simply unaware of how his body worked. He did not recognize his symptoms as guides to well-living. George was well on his way to becoming the typical medicalized citizen. Thankfully, his fiancée called him to a higher level of awareness.

Health

The assumptions of our young man, George, are the epitome of how our culture has been trained to think of health. We've learned to view "health" as the absence of disease, and indeed, as the absence of pain or suffering. Yes, at some level, most of us realize that such a state is unrealistic; and some of us are aware that the World Health Organization defines health in terms of quality of life. And yet we persist in expecting a professional to remove our bodily irritations and cause us to achieve this mythical symptom-free state. For about 50 years, Americans have been subject to the constant advertising refrain, "Please consult your doctor before making any changes" – a legal postscript that has generated a disempowered population dependent on endless professional interventions.

In 1976 a wonderful Maryland physician, Harvey Minchew, MD, invited a group of acupuncturists to speak to his medical team. After the conversation he essentially said, "I'm trained to treat an ulcer, to treat pathologies. If you bring me a tummy pain, I have to send you away with the instruction to come back when you have a real pathology – a pathology that I've been trained to treat."

Health-care Workers

Prior to the factories of the industrial revolution, there were no health-care workers. *The concept of being healthy did not exist.* Of course, everyone had symptoms. Symptoms came and went. If the symptoms got more intense and you didn't know how to deal with them on your own, there were people in the neighborhood who could help you – people who knew how to tend a cold, tend the flu, tend a fever, tend a backache, tend a headache. There were the herbalists. There were the bonesetters. There were the butchers and barbers who could do minor surgery. There was the collective wisdom of the human race, including wisdom from Hippocrates and Galen, from herbalists and the herbal wisdom tradition passed down in families. Yet people never suffered from the expectation that they should be "healthy." One was aware suffering came and went, that life included pains and aches – things one paid attention to, changing one's life pattern in order to keep living well and to keep life moving forward.

With the Industrial Revolution, the question arose as to which of the factory workers showing symptoms had to come to work and who could stay at home. Thus was invented the first health-care worker, the person assigned the task of determining which factory worker with signs of illness would get permission to take the day off; and then, immediately, the factory owners hired persons to get the ill laborers back to work as quickly as possible. Suddenly, being healthy had an economic premium of being available in the labor force.

A similar scenario played out in China in 1950 when Mao Tse-tung wanted the industrial and agricultural communes to be more effective and efficient, and not lose productivity through illness. Thus we see the invention of the "barefoot doctor," the community herbalist/acupuncturist who used forms of treatment designed to "disappear" symptoms so individuals could get back to work, not designed to guide them in learning about how to tend themselves, as much of classical Chinese medicine had wisely focused on.

The difference between learning about one's self and how to live well, and having symptoms removed in order to get back to work – that's a vast and largely unobserved chasm in the modern world.

I attribute much of the thinking in this essay to my remarkable mentor, Ivan Illich. It reflects what I have crafted from over 50 years of conversations and from reading his books, including *Medical Nemesis*.

Separation of Body and Mind

The idea of the body as a biologic system distinct from our mind, our thoughts, and our spirit has been a predicate of modern science for centuries – an idea increasingly part of our thinking since the 17th century when Descartes, called the father of modern philosophy, embedded the concept that mind and body are separate.

In a 1993 television interview, Bill Moyers asked Candace Pert – the noted biophysiologist and author who is largely responsible for our understanding of neuropeptides – about a common scientific assumption: "It's been knocking around the West a long time, the notion that the mind is somehow distinct from the body," he said. With a smile, Candace replied, "Well, that just goes back to a turf deal that Descartes made with the Roman Catholic Church. He got to study science, as we know it, and left the soul, the mind, the emotions and consciousness to the realm of the Church." [3,4] So what we are dealing with 400 years later is the end of a classic turf battle. And this turf battle has serious implications.

We all experience upsetting thoughts that have a palpable impact in our body; and this impact can be measured through blood pressure, sugar levels, and other biochemical testing. Thus we all experience evidence on a daily basis that the mind and body are connected. And yet, we continue to respect research results based on the assumption that the body and mind are separate.

We relate to a medical structure within which we take our mind to a psychologist; we take our spirit to a priest, a pastor, a rabbi, or an imam; and we take the body to a physician, a biologist, or a biochemist. These silos seldom relate to each other, and in fact, we assume they function without relevance to each other. Our modern allopathic medicine system is predicated on the body as a standardized organism with predictable interactions. But the reality is that our body, mind, and spirit are interwoven – so interwoven that it is now widely accepted that our thoughts, habits of mind, emotions, and intentions alter the chemistry of our bodies from moment to moment and affect the way chemical drugs interact with our bodies.

Over my 40 years of clinical practice, I have replaced the idea of separate silos by speaking not of body, mind, spirit, but rather of the densest part of ourselves, our bones, and the least dense part of ourselves, our breath and our thoughts – that is the spectrum. Each aspect or level of that spectrum endlessly and relentlessly impacts all of the others.

Making this shift changes the whole set of assumptions of our expert-based modern care.

Evidence-based Medicine

The idea that we should document the impact of an intervention using clinical results – evidence-based medicine, in other words – sounds reasonable, which is why it has been the mantra of the medical community for the past 40 years: The only kind of medicine that should be allowed is that which has been proven by standardized double-blind studies.

The standardized double-blind study is predicated on generating predictable results by conducting the study using participants who fit a standard set of measurements. While these participants may be slightly variable for height and weight and other observable phenomena, the study does not take into account thoughts, intentionality, and personal history.

The idea of the human body as a standardized machine was so prevalent that NIH researchers long assumed that studies on the male body provided evidence applicable to female bodies. This assumption collapsed only when the female members of the US Congress demanded separate studies for women and children.

The validity of standardized studies – the gold standard of modern medicine – becomes even more questionable if we admit the unique complexity of the biochemistry of each individual. John Ioannidis, MD, Professor of Medicine at Stanford University, has written extensively about the difficulty of the double-blind clinical trial.[5] Results of such studies frustrate the American public with contradictory messages on a daily basis: On Monday, it's okay to drink coffee because it helps the heart; on Tuesday, it's bad to drink coffee because it may be a carcinogen; on Wednesday, it prevents cancer.

Because this method became the gold standard, as a culture we've only recently begun to consider the importance of outcome-based medical practices and research – that is, medicine and research focused on the functional benefits to the patients rather than on proving the unique mechanism by which an intervention works.

I would also note an article in the December 12, 2011 issue of *The New Yorker* about the power of placebo and the importance of having a conversation about the role of the healer, the person who is interacting with the patient. This article, which draws on interviews with Ted Kaptchuk of Harvard and Wayne Jonas of the Samueli Institute, points to the insufficiency of the typical gold standard method of Western research, which excludes and does not consider patients' reports about the outcomes of their treatment.[6]

Furthermore, the question of the validity of standardized studies becomes even more complex when we admit the power of Heisenberg's uncertainty principle: The mind affects the body, the body affects the mind, and thus our body chemistry is constantly in flux and is not predictable or standardized.[7]

Payment for Procedures

A corollary of our insurance conversation and the evidence-based medicine conversation is that payments in modern American medicine are made on a per-procedure basis. Thus insurance or individuals pay for an office visit, for a drug, for a test. This focus on payment-for-procedure is radically different from ancient China where, according to lore, you paid the physician to keep you well and the physician paid you if you got sick.

This pay-for-procedure approach means no one is held accountable for the overall wellness benefit, for the outcome of the interaction. Thus, payments are linked to the questions, "Is there an identifiable disease?" and "What are the procedures that can be related to the disease?" They are not linked to benefit for the patient.

In this process, the whole person – the patient – has disappeared, and the practitioner has disappeared, as well. In philosophical terms, the instruments of action have become the center of the action, and the organism itself has vanished. The implications of this conversation are wider than we have space to discuss in this essay. However, it is critical we underscore the significance of the pay-for-procedure process in the failures of our current system.

As an acupuncturist, I'm aware of the suggestion that treatment charges be made on a per-needle basis so that payment would be related to how many needles I use. Here you can see the incentive to violate the ancient dictum of "less is more," of the law of least action, and to use many, many needles. Of course, this is absurd; and it's important we understand that when looked at from a different perspective, much of this conversation is simply nonsensical.

Stress

It's common to say we are stressed. In the early 1900s, *stress* was a term that could be applied only to machines, concrete, and steel. It was an engineering term. At that time, referring to a human being as stressed would have sounded foolish. This changed in the 1930s with the work of Hans Selye, considered the father of modern stress theory. Increasingly, human beings were labeled as "stressed." Now we take "stress" for granted in describing a person, and "stress reduction" has become a major industry.

However, what's hidden in this concept of "stress" is the shift in our understanding of the human body – a shift from a holistic being to that of a machine that can manage stress by replacing or reconditioning individual parts. In this new model, there is no room for understanding the unique manifestations of "stress" in each person's body.

Historically, the word *stress* replaced the word *grief*. Before we were "stressed" we were permitted to cry and lament the nature of the human condition. Now we are sentenced to the task of overcoming the nature of nature. Scott Peck's bestseller, *The Road Less Traveled*, begins with the words, "Life is difficult" – this does not mean that coping with difficulty needs to be a pathology.[8]

Specialization: The Body as Parts

Again, there is a long history of change from the understanding of the body as a living organism with the capacity to heal itself in union with nature, to understanding the body as a machine with parts, which is the accepted modern perspective. Because the modern body has parts, we accept without reflection the idea of medical specialization.

There is a long and well-documented history of how specialization evolved. Many people defend the idea of separate parts that can be tended separately, as did many in regard to the Cartesian separation of the mind and the body discussed above. With medical specialization, the human being takes a breathing problem to one specialist, and a problem with urine to another specialist. These specialists may have no idea about the whole person, no idea what other specialists are doing, no access to what might be going on in the world of thought, emotional change, or social conflict.

In a previous essay I used the example of a patient referred to me by an internist worried that she was now seeing five specialists: a pulmonary specialist, a urinary specialist, an orthopedic specialist, a gastroenterological specialist, and a gynecologist. The internist was concerned about interactions among the medications prescribed by these five specialists, and indeed, concerned that the patient was not getting better. As you may recall, I looked at the patient from a different perspective and observed that the lower part of her abdomen, the focus of four of the five specialists, was very cold; and the upper part of her abdomen, where one of the specialists was focused, was very hot. When she was taught deep breathing, which brought warmth deeper into her body and supported patterns of eating that enhanced warmth, she, herself, addressed this imbalance; and the need for the specialists shifted.

Victimhood and the Professionalization of Life

Individuals quickly can become patients with disease labels, and those patients quickly become victims of the disease that has

mysteriously happened to them and over which they are power-
less. Something completely external has happened to their body
machine, and thus they are a victim – much as anyone can become
the victim of a crime or an accident. Many then join communities
in order to experience belonging and support. This is the process by
which we transform from unique individuals into Cancer Survivors,
Arthritic Persons, Asthma Sufferers, etc.

In the world that focuses on separate parts, the individual becomes a victim to something that has invaded, stressed, or troubled
a particular part of the body. The victim, who goes to the expert in
fixing that part, is allowed not to be responsible for any part of the
problem. Of course, this is not to say a specialist may not have a
role in repairing muscles or a broken bone, or in helping to rectify
some internal problem. However, the moment we become the pow-
erless, irresponsible victim, we are no longer the individual with
the innate healing power of a natural organism. Thus, the process
becomes dismayingly depersonalized and disempowering.

John McKnight from Northwestern University in Chicago
made a presentation titled "John Deere and the Bereavement
Counselor" at the 1984 Schumacher Society Lecture Series, where
he emphasized that in earlier times when someone died in a
Midwestern community, the neighbors gathered around and tended the family. They brought food, grieved and laughed together,
and created the funeral. But times have changed. In the modern
world the neighbors are looking out the window at the house of
the bereaved, waiting until the grief counselor has come and gone,
because no one would assume that they knew how to tend life in
a moment of grief as well as the professional grief counselor. This
image is emblematic of how life has changed, a reminder of the
transformation of an organic and harmonious world to one of de-
personalization and professionalization.[9]

We've pointed to the professionalization of dying and death.
Now we have professionalization of many other aspects of our

everyday life, including how we eat and how we exercise. We need a nutritionist to work with us in choosing food. We no longer consider ourselves capable of knowing, as does every animal on the planet, what food to eat based on its smell, its flavor, and the impact it has on our body. And we need a professional trainer: We no longer know how to exercise and move our bodies on a daily basis without the intervention of a professional. We have disconnected from our inner wisdom.

Medicalization

What has happened to childbirth is an illuminating example of medicalization. Childbirth used to be a community activity tended by the women. I understand childbirth has its dangers: My own mother died in childbirth while giving birth to a baby who would have been my younger sister if she had not also died. It's highly likely my mother died from an infection contracted in the hospital rather than from a direct complication of childbirth – I will never know.

According to the Harvard Kennedy School Review, data collected in the mid-1990s indicate that the highest rate of infant survival in the United States was among poor Hispanic women in South Texas who had no access to health care. In other words, the most successful childbirth outcomes in the United States were where there was no medical intervention. It is very interesting that the United States has a relatively low maternal and infant survival rate as compared to other developed nations where there is less intense medicalization of childbirth.[10]

In the United States, we now tend to medicalize virtually everything. If we have a concern about our health, we hear the mantra of the past 40 years, "Please see your doctor." And when we go to the doctor, if he suspects that what he sees is something normal and passing, he's virtually not allowed to say that to us without running a battery of tests, which become more and more expensive. So even if the real reason you're having symptoms is that you're not getting enough sleep or that you're drinking too much caffeine, he may not have enough time with you to make that discovery; yet he will write referrals for batteries of tests which, in the vast majority of cases, will show that you have nothing wrong.

Even with a risk-benefit ratio indicating very little risk, health professionals will protect themselves from making the slightest error and order the tests. Human life has become medicalized. I see many patients who are unable to describe their own symptoms, how they feel in their own bodies – they tell me what the doctor has told them from a test.

Prevention

Prevention seems like a wonderful concept: We will prevent the diseases that will happen in the future. However in doing this, we often stop living in the present and start a fight with life. There is documentation that runners who run every day to prevent a heart attack in the future actually spend more time running than their life is extended by the prevention of a heart attack. Thus the activity of running for the sake of preventing a future event is actually counterproductive in terms of the amount of time available to be with family and friends and to experience the fullness of life.

Most of what we call "prevention" and what we fund as prevention is not actually prevention; it is early detection of the disease. It may be that we are now detecting diseases with more and more sophisticated mammography and other tests, finding more and more minor cancerous cells which, in fact, the body itself would have sloughed off, given its own devices. But the moment the cell is detected, it becomes a "disease" with all the complications and trauma and shock that accompany the process.

In US Senate testimony in February 2009, many examples were cited pointing to the fact that real-time benefits were much more effective in developing daily habits for living well than was fear-based advertising.[11]

Years ago, a woman in her forties came to my office in shock and tears that she had been diagnosed with osteoporosis. This diagnosis began to govern her life at age 40 because she was terrified of what would happen to her bones as she got into her sixties, seventies, and eighties. She began to design her life around the medications and drugs needed to prevent any worsening of her disease. Loss of bone mass – something that couldn't have been measured more than 20 years ago – is not to be belittled and needs to be addressed. However, beyond medications, there are numerous effective ways to address bone loss and bone breaks. It's well documented that doing tai chi and living well every day greatly reduces bone breaks in the elderly. Activities that cultivate our well-being and bring pleasure and satisfaction to life are our best medicine – preventive and healing activities that bring real-time payoff such as sleep and rest, deep breathing, running and walking, eating well, time with friends, and tai chi.

Health Insurance – What Is It, and What Should It Pay For?

A big sticking point in the health-care debate is health insurance because it is a concept widely misunderstood by the majority of Americans. While most of us think of "insurance" as something that pays for the sudden consequences of an unforeseen event – such as we might expect from home or auto insurance – most of what we call health insurance is a system in which our employer or the government pays the cost of our regular health care. This sort of health plan usually is provided under the auspices of an insurance company like Blue Cross; however, most often the actual expense is borne by the large corporation that employs you or by the government. The insurance company is acting on behalf of the corporation or government in tracking details and payments. For this, the "insurer" is paid a fee per transaction. This is not what is usually thought of as insurance. This is simply a method of paying for agreed-upon services.

A small percentage of the population is covered by *real* insurance policies, in which individuals pool their premiums with an insurance company against their shared risk of illness. They pay these premiums directly out of their own pockets; and the insurance companies – the Blues, Kaiser, Connecticut General – take on the balance of risk for those individuals. The cost of that type of insurance, real "insurance," is now astronomical, especially for someone with a preexisting condition. Most insurance companies carefully "cherry pick" whom they will allow into such policies in order to minimize the risk of having to pay anything. It is in this system where you find controversies, for example, about "What is a preexisting condition?" and about coverage suddenly being dropped in the presence of large claims.

The majority of us who are lucky enough to be insured are covered by one of these large plans in which our regular health-care expenses are paid for by our employer (or the government through Medicare and Medicaid); and this can be a seemingly endless expense item because almost anything can be connected to health care. My organic food and my athletic club membership help me feel well. And what about the round of golf that lets me release all that stress? And my theater tickets? Yoga class? Shouldn't they be paid for by my health insurance? What are the limits on the expenditure we call health care? Where is the margin between what is a health-care cost and what is the cost of the general sustenance of a life well lived? Where does it make sense for health plans to intervene earlier in ways that don't look like traditional health care but save money for everyone in the long run?

One of the ways the insurance industry is attempting to limit health-care expenses is by mandating that everyone who requests payment present their claim in terms of a covered disease. There must be a diagnosis – early detection of a diagnosed disease, prevention of a diagnosed disease. We must be in some sort of conversation about disease in order to access health-care or health-insurance payments. Thus it is logical to keep expanding the range of what is defined as "disease"; and there is much financial benefit if the normal sufferings of life can be transformed into a diagnosis. New disease labels are being created all the time, as are new drugs and machines to combat those disease labels (although in many cases the intervention is created before the disease).

Malpractice Insurance, Tort Reform, and Risk

As we seek to avoid suffering and death at all costs, endlessly increasing the price of professionalized care, we also demand such care be risk free – perfect and without error every time. This is an inhuman demand that corresponds to our inhuman desire/expectation that there be no death and suffering.

It is reported that malpractice suits add significantly to the cost of health care, a cost often cited as perhaps up to two percent of total health-care expenditures. To me, this seems a relatively proportionate cost in our huge health-care system and a genuine protection against negligence and incompetence. However, the real cost of our effort to avoid all risks is not the cost of the lawsuits, legal fees, and payments for mistakes and errors. The real cost is the fear engendered in professionals as they attempt to be error-free superheroes and thus order endless tests at great expense – tests that otherwise might not be ordered and actually are rarely needed.

A risk-adverse life is not really living. It is an existence mired in fear; and it is extremely expensive for all of us.

NOTES

1. Ezekiel J. Emanuel and Jeffrey B. Liebman, "The End of Health Insurance Companies." *New York Times* Opinionator Online Commentary (January 30, 2012). Ezekiel Emanuel, a bioethicist who has served at the National Institutes of Health, is currently Vice Provost, University of Pennsylvania. Jeffrey Liebman is currently Executive Associate Director of the Office of Management and Budget, and formerly Professor of Public Policy at Harvard University.

2. Nortin Hadler, *The Last Well Person: How to Stay Well Despite the Health-Care System* (McGill-Queen's University Press. April 2004).

3. Bill Moyers, *Healing and the Mind*, Companion Volume to Bill Moyers' PBS TV Series (Main Street Books, 1995).

4. Candace B. Pert, *Molecules Of Emotion: The Science Behind Mind-Body Medicine* (Simon & Schuster, 1999).

5. For a list of John Ioannidis's publications, see his academic profile on the Stanford School of Medicine website, med.stanford.edu/profiles. Also see:
    – Sharon Begley, "Why Almost Everything You Hear About Medicine is Wrong." *Newsweek* (January 24, 2011).
    – Sharon Begley, *Train Your Mind, Change Your Brain: How a New Science Reveals Our Extraordinary Potential to Transform Ourselves* (Ballantine Books, 2007).

6. Michael Specter, "The Power of Nothing: Could studying the placebo effect change the way we think about medicine?" *The New Yorker* (December 12, 2011).

7. This expression of Heisenberg's uncertainty principle is based on what I have learned from physicist Hans-Peter Dürr in his lectures and seminars at Tai Sophia Institute. Hans-Peter was Heisenberg's main assistant for almost 20 years and served as executive director of the Max Planck Institute.

8. Much of this thinking around stress I have derived from my understanding of the writings of Robert Kugelman of the University of Dallas, and from conversations with Robert Kugelman and Ivan Illich. I give credit to them; and my expression of what I've learned from them is entirely mine.

9. John L. McKnight's presentation at the Fourth Annual E. F. Schumacher Society Lecture Series is available online at www.schumachersociety.org. His talk, titled "John Deere and the Bereavement Counselor," is also available in pamphlet form at the Schumacher website.

10. See "The Demand Side of the Health Care Crisis," a 1993 interview with Ronald David, MD, of Harvard's John F. Kennedy School of Government. The interview, originally published in *Harvard Magazine*, is available in *Meridians*, Late Summer 1993.

11. Full testimony presented before the US Senate Committee on Health, Education, Labor, and Pensions at the February 2009 hearing titled "Principles of Integrative Health: A Path to Health Care Reform" can be accessed at www.help.senate.gov.

We Are at War *with* Our Bodies

"All sickness is homesickness."
– Dianne Connelly

I WAS TEACHING a class at the University of Pennsylvania School of Medicine, mainly second-year medical students. As part of the course, I had the students keep a journal of the symptoms that come and go in their lives day-to-day, from headaches to stomachaches to sleeplessness to whatever they observed. Each week at the start of the class we would discuss what they had learned from, and about, their symptoms.

This was a new exercise for the students. Many of them became angry when they realized that although they were scientists, they never had learned to apply their scientific observations to their own bodily functions – that was pretty disturbing to them.

About four weeks in, a student said that in the previous week he had come to class exhausted and tired from a very stressful day, and that at the end of the evening there was an unexpected storm. As he bicycled home, upset and in the rain, he was ruining a new shirt – and he got lost. By the time he reached home, he was enraged. He began to speak loudly and express his anger to his housemates. Finally, the rage turned into uncontrollable sobbing.

Then he said to us, "What you don't know is that during the summer I began to feel a lump in my throat; and the lump began to grow and bother me so much so that I went to my physician asking how I could treat it. The physician was totally puzzled and referred me to a surgeon. I met with the surgeon recently, and we discussed possible surgeries that would remove this lump and tension from my throat." Then, the student said, something amazing happened. After a night of upset and crying, he woke up in the morning with no lump in his throat for the first time in four or five months. "Now," he said, "I realize that whenever I have tension, there is a pulling in my throat."

Are we at war? Or are we living in possibility? A recent issue of the *Baltimore Sun* had a banner headline about what is happening with the drug buprenorphine, which has been promoted in Baltimore and across the United States as a great contribution to the *war* on drugs. It is supposed to be a simple way to have people come off illicit recreational drugs; and now, as with methadone, it is becoming a street drug for sale. Some of the ammunition in the war on drugs contributes to the worsening of that war.

My friend, Al Duha Chase, had been a drug dealer in Baltimore and had spent time in prison. By the time I knew him, however, he had trained himself as a remarkable tai chi teacher. His explanation for his years-long addiction: "Heroin is a wonderful friend. If you take me off my heroin, you better build me a friendship community." Are we in a war on drugs? Or are drugs the sign of our deep longing for belonging, for community, for relationships?

I read an article recently about our food chain, about how vast amounts of antibiotics are used in the industrial production of pork. Our pig farms may be a big source of antibiotic-resistant forms of staphylococcus, which are causing 100,000 illnesses a year and

19,000 deaths – more deaths than caused by AIDS. We have a war on the bacteria, which respond by growing and evolving. The Food and Drug Administration has warned parents of young children to limit the use of antibiotics and over-the-counter medications for colds. The war on the colds was building a resistance in microorganisms that created more difficulty than benefit for our children.[1]

When we fight death, when we fight suffering and illness, we actually may be enhancing the force of illness. War breeds war.

If we look at the expense rates for our health-care system in the United States, we find costs that resemble the costs of fighting a literal war, with the aggressive policies to match. We are fighting a war on drug addiction, addiction to drugs both legally prescribed and illegally obtained; we are fighting a war on smoking; we are fighting a war on obesity; we are fighting a war on diabetes; we are fighting wars on various cancers; we are fighting a war on heart disease. I could go on and on. And beyond all of this, we are fighting a war about this system that we call health care.

It seems clear to me that humans must learn to live in harmony with forces of nature (and with each other) rather than wage counterproductive battles in opposition to those forces. In *The Extraordinary Healing Power of Ordinary Things*, Larry Dossey describes how children who grow up in households that are kept antiseptically clean are much more susceptible to infections than children who grow up eating the requisite "pound of dirt," which was the conversation understood by my simple immigrant parents.[2]

These wars against what is natural are a symptom that we are afraid of the texture of life itself. And out-of-control fear is also an illness, one that blinds us to other possibilities.

It is well understood that many of the popular disease labels have their roots in stress and in inflammation. Even if we were to win the wars and rid the person of these particular diseases, there's the question as to whether we can reduce the stress – the root of the issue – so the person's immune system will have a stronger natural ability to cope with whatever becomes the next disease, the next war. The dilemma is that we are so accustomed to having a war with our problems that we have no idea what else we might do, and whether the alternatives might bring greater benefits for living.

In 1970 an extraordinary physician, Harvey Minchew, MD, in Maryland's Howard County founded the first HMO in the United States outside of the Kaiser Permanente HMO in California. Shortly after we opened an acupuncture center in Columbia, Maryland, in the fall of 1975, he invited us to speak with the staff of the Columbia Medical Plan. At that time, it was a courageous invitation! He made an important statement at the end of that meeting: "I'm highly trained to deal with an ulcer," he said. "But I was never taught what to do with a tummy pain before it became an ulcer. So I have to wait until we have a pathology before I'm able to deal with it." Then he said to us, "If you know something about dealing with a tummy pain before it becomes a disease, go for it."

When we name the disease, we are setting up the battle lines for a war against the disease; but this pioneering physician's wisdom avoids that paradigm. In the noise of the modern world, we have stopped paying attention to the minor signs given by our own body before they become major signs, before they become pathologies that stop our bodies. Think in terms of the modern warning system in a car that lets you know when a door isn't fully closed. When I was younger, other drivers would honk and wave and point to your door; and if you were at a stoplight, they would roll down their windows and tell you. It was personal and direct.

After over 30 years of collecting the words of patients, my colleagues and I know that there is the potential for empowered living, for something besides war. People who come in with a migraine don't report we "cured" their migraine. They say, "You know, I notice it starts several days before it gets to be a migraine. Usually I have a little funny feeling in my lower back. If I pay attention to that funny feeling, either by resting or by getting exercise or whatever my body has been lacking, I rarely, if ever, get a migraine." In other words, the body has a warning system based on minor symptoms, which gives us the possibility of not going to war.

We are very accustomed to the early warning system in our car where a series of lights tell us at an early stage, before there is breakdown, if our car needs tending. The same principle applies to our body: By paying attention to the minor signs, we open ourselves to the possibility of avoiding war with our body and of living in harmony with our body's wisdom.

I say patients have been trained to bring a "ticket" to a doctor's office. They need to bring something of significant import that a doctor has been trained to pay attention to, because doctors trained in the modern world basically have only a few options: find a pathology, keep testing until they find a pathology, send you home and wait for a pathology to develop, or engage you in all sorts of preventive activities – activities we assume have a life-saving cost-benefit ratio, but often, we're finding, do not.

On the rare occasion when I'm in a doctor's office as a patient, I will mention minor symptoms – and I see the doctor's eyes glaze over. I know those symptoms are related to other things and I need to pay attention to them, but the doctor is not trained to ask the series of questions that may lead to those "other things" and help me learn. Without an obvious need, I have no ticket to bring to the doctor.

I do have my wonderful left ankle that aches whenever I'm not paying attention to rest or food or tensions in my body. I've learned over the years that my left ankle is my best teacher. To illustrate the importance of paying attention to our symptoms, I'll repeat a story: More than 20 years ago I first learned this lesson from Charlie, who told me, "Asthma has become my friend. Now, when I begin that minor wheezing, I pay attention and take care of myself, and I avoid going to the emergency room or going on heavy medications."

I wrote in *Common Sense for the Healing Arts* about visiting four treatment rooms in a row, where I talked with highly educated people, none of whom could describe the sensations in his/her body; they could only tell me what doctors had said to them about their diseases.[3] They had obliterated their aches and pains with medications or by pushing through them. They came to me saying, "I have arthritis." And if I said, "How do you know?" they replied, "The doctor told me." "How does the doctor know?" I asked. "He did tests," they said. Then I pointed out to these clients that they already knew that their body was in trouble; they knew the symptoms of heat, cold, pain – symptoms coming and going, depending on the client's activities. The doctor had put a label on those symptoms, overriding what they already knew. I told them this was a way they lose their power: they ignore their body's wisdom and turn over the possibility of wellness to an "expert."

We have been taught over the past 50 years to ignore, override, or obliterate the sensations of our body until, out of desperation, they reach the level of pathology. We now bypass bodily sensations and ignore our body's intelligence/wisdom, which in the past would have guided us in how to live well and in harmony with nature.

If we are not at war, then what is the possibility? Many possibilities are discussed more widely in Essay 9.

The Art of Living Foundation, started by a wise teacher, Ravi Shankar of India, now has educational projects in more than a hundred countries. When he saw learning difficulties, he saw possibility instead of problem. When he saw children who didn't know how to breathe well, never mind know their ABCs or math, he began to teach them a very simplified form of yoga and breathing exercises. He brought the program to schools throughout the world, and now many young school children start their school day with these simple exercises. In the schools where children participate in the program, learning scores have increased.

My friend Nortin Hadler, whom I've cited elsewhere, assumes humans have the ability to pay attention to their body, and if they pay attention to the wisdom of their body – and more importantly, if they learn from it and adjust their ways of living – they will achieve an age of at least 85, which he calls their birthright. The one place where Nortin and I disagree is that I no longer observe that the healthiest of human beings have access to that inner wisdom. Instead, they have access to their medical records and the results of tests their doctors have ordered and used to analyze their worsening symptoms.[4]

Accessing the body's wisdom – this is the major work that must be done if we are to reduce health-care costs, thus freeing up funds to assure that those who do have a serious pathology can access quality treatment.

NOTES

1. Michael Pollan, *The Omnivore's Dilemma: A Natural History of Four Meals* (Penguin, 2007).

2. Larry Dossey, *The Extraordinary Healing Power of Ordinary Things: Fourteen Natural Steps to Health and Happiness* (Three Rivers Press, 2007).

3. Robert M. Duggan, *Common Sense for the Healing Arts* (Tai Sophia Press, 2003).

4. Nortin Hadler, *The Last Well Person: How to Stay Well Despite the Health-Care System* (McGill-Queen's University Press, May 2004). *Worried Sick: A Prescription for Health in an Overtreated America* (University of North Carolina Press, 2008).

Economics 101 –
It Can't Work This Way

*When asked, "What thing about humanity surprises you
the most?" the Dalai Lama answered: "Man . . . Because he
sacrifices his health in order to make money. Then he sacrifices
money to recuperate his health. And then he is so anxious about
the future that he does not enjoy the present, the result being that
he does not live in the present or the future; he lives as if he is
never going to die, and then dies having never really lived."*
*– Although the origin is uncertain, this quote is widely attributed
to the Dalai Lama XIV.*

THE CONUNDRUM OF the cost-quality-access triangle by now might sound like a familiar catch-22: If you increase *access* to health care, you necessarily increase its *costs*, reducing *quality* because financing can't be sustained at that level. If your desire is to increase quality, you can do it only by reducing access or adding those unsustainable costs. Reducing access will lead to a public outcry of rationing, which makes that option politically unsustainable. Yet the reality is that we already ration access, limit quality, and attempt to limit costs with disastrous results (as illustrated in previous essays).

While cost-quality-access is widely accepted as an unbreakable conundrum, it is actually a false one. Most individuals accessing the system do not have the health issues that the system is optimized to tend. It's been estimated that $1.2 trillion of the current annual US health-care costs are wasted because patient complaints are related to their lifestyle, and thus not responsive to the type of intervention the health system is prepared to provide.

The fallacy of the cost-quality-access triangle is illustrated by a Howard County Chamber of Commerce presentation I attended a few years ago. The speaker, a public health doctor, was discussing the cost to businesses' bottom lines of the most costly and most common chronic diseases – diabetes, heart disease, arthritis, obesity – and initiated the conversation with the usual questions: "How do we treat the disease? How do we give everyone access to treatment? How do we pay for all of this?" She pointed out that none of the cost was necessary, that all of these diseases are, at their common root, inflammatory stress responses. "Your workplaces are inflamed," she said. "When you change the stress in your workplaces, you will not have these costs on your bottom line." The speaker's invitation, for those who could hear it, was to discover a financial benefit for their corporation's bottom line in the simple act of being nice to their employees.

Corporations and the Funding of Care in the USA

"If this goes on another 10 years, the only employees in Cincinnati will either be working for the hospitals, or lawyers suing the hospitals, or lawyers defending the hospitals."

– Jeffrey Immelt, GE Chairman and Chief Executive Officer,

"Economics 101"

at a gathering of Cincinnati-area business leaders (Cincinnati Enquirer, *February 27, 2010)*

For a variety of historical reasons mostly related to wage controls during World War II, a significant portion of the burden of health-care costs in the United States, unlike most of the world, has been placed on our corporations. With a medical system that focuses on separate diseases and rarely takes into account the whole person, our American corporations carry very significant costs that in other countries would be covered by the public tax system – and this skews the cost structures of operating a business in the US as well as the salary systems for employees.

I was traveling from Baltimore to New York on Amtrak in 2009 when I overheard a group of Amtrak employees in the next booth discussing the financial collapse of General Motors. These ordinary citizens clearly understood that a good part of that collapse was due to the impossibility of a company carrying the total health-care costs for current and past employees, echoing the long-recognized fact that the cost of health care for employees who made the car was greater than the cost of the steel they used in making the car. And they understood this structure is very bad for our economy – it goes beyond health care, affecting every aspect of the American economic and industrial life.

We're talking about an essentially unlimited expense related to the expectations of preventing death and suffering, which – in an unexamined, unquestioned, and truly irrational way – now appears as an ordinary and expected expense on the accounts of these corporations. In recent years many of these costs have been transferred back to the worker to be paid out-of-pocket, building political pressure to "do something" about the health-insurance system. And yet, underneath all the shifting and bargaining and angst about costs lies the question: "Is there any limit to that cost structure?" In the economics conversation about the cost-quality-access triangle, we are in an unsolvable bind. As long as the objective of health care is to prevent death and all suffering, the costs will continue to escalate; and thus the bottom-line budgets of government and corporations (and increasingly of citizens, as health-care costs shift to them) will continue to spiral out of control.

There is an alternative conversation, one in which people learn how the real-time benefits of living well are radically different and much less expensive. This alternative conversation promotes the experience of our bodily symptoms as teachers rather than as problems to be turned over to experts. It is very much in the interest of corporate leaders to create the radical transformations necessary to begin this alternative conversation in an effective way, so that these efforts will be picked up and copied by the government.

Government Cash and Escalating Health-care Costs

The government health-care program of Medicare and Medicaid is essentially a single-payer system with complex regulations – regulations that again define the world of health care with diagnoses and procedures, not by benefit to the whole person, and (for the purposes of this conversation) with no way to contain costs or restrict access while also under great political pressure to increase quality. Whatever seems medically effective must be covered by these plans, regardless of costs. This system can be simplified and streamlined; but I'm not sure electronic records would be the panacea in a health-care culture where the greatest patient complaint is that nobody listens, and where the key issues in the most expensive cases seem to be related to lifestyle issues – issues that disappear amid the categories of electronic data-sorting.

When it comes to government coverage, it will be very difficult to limit costs through political action alone; the normal course of political activity is to expand coverage. That is why corporate experiments are very important in demonstrating the effectiveness of wellness-based economics, of the delivery of wellness packages where the individual has a sense of satisfaction and well-being as well as a sense of the potential dangers of medicalized interventions.

In agreement with other responsible observers, I believe government health-care spending will continue to overwhelm our economy as the number of elderly citizens increases, and as the costs of high-tech care continue to spiral, along with other expensive attempts at preventing death and suffering. Politically, there will be no way to contain those costs. Ivan Illich made an observation that speaks directly to what we're experiencing: "A culture that attempts to prevent death and disease will spend itself out of existence in that effort."

Hidden Dollars: Economics of the Emergency Room and the Uninsured

Although approximately 49 to 50 million Americans are uninsured at the moment, these individuals do receive urgent and emergency care, thanks to payments from the rest of us. No one is turned away and allowed to die unnecessarily, at least not yet. In Maryland, for example, a percentage of funds from all insurers is allocated by a very complex system to every hospital for the emergency care of the uninsured. Everyone gets coverage, but it is in the least effective way possible. No rational person would have designed the existing system from scratch. The uninsured can get emergency care, but they cannot access the system at a wellness level, a prevention level, or even a routine symptom level; they must wait until their symptoms escalate to the point of expensive pathology. In our present system we reimburse for a heart transplant and for a long hospitalization for pneumonia; but we will not reimburse for the aspirin that might have prevented a heart condition, nor for the wellness education that might have led the person with pneumonia to stop eating excess dairy long before the congestion escalated to a serious infection. Thus we are in a bind. The money is at the hospitals waiting to be spent on cutting-edge technology; if those funds could be transferred to the earlier stage, there would be plenty of money to cover the uninsured before their conditions reach an emergency level.

If you examine how this process is working in inner city neighborhoods, it's clear that when it's wintertime and residents are cold with no place to go, they understand what symptoms they need to appear to have so they can gain admission to the ER, and eventually, to a hospital room for several nights. I've heard people teach others how to do this. In truth, many of these fabricated symptoms would be treated much more effectively through lifestyle changes than in the ER. All of us are paying for these inefficiencies.

Unnecessary Use of the Primary Care Doctor

Another indication of how costs are distorted is revealed in data showing that 70 percent of visits to doctors in the United States are for functional disorders and symptoms for which there is no pathology – for example, "I'm depressed and tired." If time were allowed for questioning and listening, the doctor likely would discover a person who doesn't exercise, drinks large amounts of caffeinated beverages, sleeps only five hours a night, and expects an MD to make him/her functional. A *functional disorder*, as distinct from a pathology, is a symptom generated by lifestyle.

Functional disorders are the result of poor diet, poor sleep, and a number of other lifestyle habits and choices. When such a case is presented to a doctor, he or she becomes frustrated because physicians have not been trained to do anything in these cases other than to say, in essence, "Take two aspirin and call me tomorrow," or more frequently, "Take this [expensive] prescription and call me in a week." And of course, when pharmaceuticals are introduced for a functional disorder, the complications (and costs) have magnified because of the danger of side effects and interactions.

Unnecessary Extension of Suffering at the End of Life

Finally, we point to the huge cost of postponing death in the last six months of life. In Essay 1, I told the story of Larry, who when confronted with the reality his life was near its end, and when told his life could be extended for perhaps six months through intensive hospital-based care, chose to have a shorter life of much higher quality with his family – a choice that saved Larry his dignity and saved all of us our portion of the hundreds of thousands of dollars for this intervention that would have been covered by Medicare.

Data about these costs vary widely, including estimates that costs for end-of-life care consume 25 percent of the health-care budget of the United States. Let's assume that only 10 percent of our total health-care expenditure is spent in the last months of life, and then assume that half of that amount would be useful in treating those who initially were given a good prospect of recovery and were not ready for death. Based on these assumptions, allowing people who are ready to die – and those for whom death is clearly imminent – to die more peacefully without traumatic intervention might save more than $100 billion per year.[1]

Yet this doesn't happen. Are we determined to preserve every moment of life at all costs, regardless of the poor quality of the person's life and the extended suffering the intervention causes the person (and their family)? In 40 years of practice, only twice have I met individuals who wanted more time regardless of the associated pain and suffering. Much more often there are cases like that of my father-in-law, who, because he was a nice man, agreed to a surgery that prevented him from dying peacefully. During the last six months of his life, he had feeding tubes in his mouth and could not speak; he could only wink and nod at us until he died.

There is nothing in this essay that everyone does not already know. However, often we don't marry these specific conversations about health care and health insurance to the issue of containing costs. As with many issues in life, the assumptions dwell in our consciousness in silos; there's no forum in which these conversations occur in one place. That's the purpose of this essay and this book – to bring together our assumptions and conversations and engender productive change.

Elimination of Waste and Inefficiency

It is possible to streamline and make Western medical care more effective and efficient. It is possible to deliver the right drug to the right patient. It is possible to enhance the experience of doctors and nurses in the health-care system. It is possible to improve all of these aspects of health care.

However, we will not change the basic cost structures of American health care until we shift the way we deal with the delayed care of acute events, chronic illnesses, functional symptoms, and the ideas of suffering and death. These aspects of the medical system account for approximately $1.2 trillion in wasted health-care expenses. Even if you assume this figure is grossly exaggerated and reduce it by 50 percent, that means at least $600 billion of wasted expenditures, which if saved through a shift in our approach to health care, would bring us in line with most other industrialized countries, dropping the amount spent on health care in the US from about 16 percent to 10 percent of the gross domestic product.

Common Sense – Where the Dollars Are

A number of years ago, a wonderful internist in Howard County, Maryland, Gary Millis, MD, started a clinic to serve individuals who did not have access to health care. The clinic was set up with the support of many local physicians and community organizations. Several evenings a week, people in need of health services could see a nurse practitioner who would tend them immediately or, if need be, refer them to other volunteers for more intensive care, including surgery or hospital-based treatment. The time with the nurse practitioner was the guide for the next steps of care.

Many uninsured in the county took advantage of this service; and obviously, the emergency room benefited when folks went to this clinic instead of to the hospital. The clinic's volunteers saved the hospital and its owner, the Johns Hopkins Hospital System, millions of dollars – dollars that went somewhere else, but not to support more of that kind of effective service. No one had the willingness to close the circle of what I call common sense.

While the service was being offered, several Tai Sophia students, including my wife, Susan, volunteered at the clinic to spend time with these clients while they were waiting to see the nurse practitioners. It became obvious to Susan and the other volunteers that this personal conversation – a form of wellness coaching – had a dramatic impact. Whether individuals came with a chronic condition or an acute situation that had just erupted, very often what had brought them to the clinic for their eight minutes of urgent care had to do with the issues of lifestyle, food, and simple misunderstandings of how to manage everyday events.

The clinic was providing the best of medical care in a brief window of contact. Costs were reduced because volunteers provided service; and the service provided access to many individuals who otherwise would have no care unless they went to an emergency room. However, the basic problem continued: the seemingly unbreakable triangle of cost-quality-access.

In that setting, there was insufficient time for the sort of dialogue and listening where the nurse or the physician could explore with patients and gain the context for the symptoms that had brought them to the clinic. The patients got limited *access,* but the *quality* of care was limited because of *costs.* In such situations, while the system costs are reduced because the visits are brief, future health-care costs will rise because individuals are not sufficiently educated to care for themselves through a healthy lifestyle and thus avoid further costly urgent care. The Tai Sophia volunteer wellness coaches, while appreciated as a nice add-on, were not appreciated as the key to breaking the triangle, and thus were not strongly encouraged to become part of the solution. The delivery of acute services is critical in health care. Yet if we deliver *only* acute service, we virtually guarantee repeated frequent visits because people have been left disempowered and dependent on an expert to fix their body when it breaks down.

An additional observation of this model is that lunch and dinner were provided for the volunteer staff and visitors by pharmaceutical representatives, who were constantly delivering gifts and free samples of medications as well as support in the form of meals – all well intentioned. However, these gifts from the pharmaceutical companies put a premium on access to medications rather than on self-awareness or self-care.

This model illustrates the "iron triangle" conundrum: We tend people only after the body has broken down; and we barely have time to provide a high quality of care because of high cost, with much of that cost due to high-tech expenses. When we do deliver preventive education – preventing heart disease, preventing cancer, preventing diabetes – it often doesn't result in the real-time payoff in behavior that prevents the heart attack, cancer, or severe diabetes in the long term. In breakdown situations, generated by fear, people often respond by making New Year's Eve-type resolutions to adopt a healthy lifestyle; then, very quickly, those resolutions for healthy behavior disappear in the busyness of everyday life, and the disease is not prevented.

For true long-term prevention, we must develop a quality delivery system that insures real-time payoffs for changes in behavior: I exercise, not just to prevent heart disease 30 years from now, but because I feel good at the end of the day. I eat better, not just to avoid obesity, but because I'm being mindful of the food I'm eating and enjoying it, and I don't feel overfilled. And I'm mindful that, in doing these things, I can keep myself out of the medicalized system.

Health-care policymakers have to face the choice: Are we educating the public only for long-term prevention of disease? Or are we educating people for an immediate, short-term benefit that also brings a great reduction in the likelihood of a long-term disease? We must design our educational programs to encourage the short-term responses individuals need and give them immediate benefit, and also guide them in learning to live well and enjoy the real-time benefit of their healthy behavior. These are the responses that reduce immediate dollar costs and at the same time reduce the long-term incidence of disease.

Again, I echo the comments of the public-health doctor mentioned in the opening paragraphs of this essay. She pointed out to the employers in the audience: "You really have a choice. You can pay to reduce the inflammation by paying for disease-care costs – for the high hospital costs, high-tech interventions, specialists, pharmaceuticals. Or you can reduce inflammation in the workplace by changing the way the workplace functions. That way you reduce stress and inflammation at work, and this provides an immediate payoff for your employees. They feel better from being tended, being paid attention to. And your health-care costs are dramatically reduced." We have examples that illustrate what she was saying, one of them in a Maryland hospital where small behavioral changes instituted by staff nurses cut the nurse turnover rates an astounding amount, saving the hospital probably more than a half-million dollars on one unit in the first year. (Each nurse turnover costs in excess of $45,000.)

Employers benefit when they create a healthier workplace – individuals who may be on the verge of getting a disease and taking days off, or who might be on the verge of a major breakdown, are less likely to get seriously ill or to have any illness at all. The immediate benefits include higher employee retention and productivity, higher employee satisfaction and enthusiasm, and higher employee wellness, resulting immediately in lower short-term medical costs. And a healthier workplace not only provides financial savings for the employers, it reduces costs to the wider society.

Where do we focus our health-care dollars? The answer matters, because health care and wellness depends on how we use those dollars. To examine this question I propose a continuum model of health care in contrast to the iron triangle of cost-access-quality, which becomes unbreakable when we focus on disease. (See diagram.)

We usually intervene at the level of "symptoms as problems," but if we don't tend the person's symptom at the problem level, it often becomes a disease.

Most physicians are highly skilled at intervening when a symptom has become a disease, but not skilled in dealing with symptoms before they reach the disease level – a very expensive point to begin intervention. In order to reduce costs and shift the conversation, we must focus on changing the point of intervention. Instead of waiting until we reach the disease level, we can pay attention to our early symptoms and use them as teachers and guides. The result will be less disease, less cost, and of course, fewer invasive interventions. We can use acupuncture before Prednisone, for example; chiropractic before surgery; yoga before fertility drugs; herbs for minor depression before Prozac for major depression; and use lifestyle training for overall well-being, as described by Andrew Weil

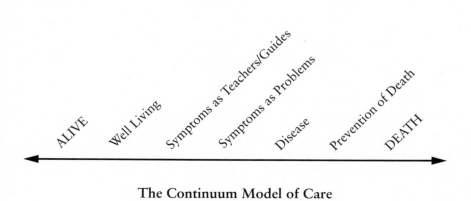

The Continuum Model of Care

in *Eight Weeks to Optimal Health* and John Travis in *The Wellness Workbook*.[2,3]

Complementary medicine is not necessarily the magic wand for this shift in health care because, like Western medicine, complementary medicine can be invasive or noninvasive; it can generate dependency or it can empower the individual. If it is following the medical model, the practitioner waits until the disease is present and then uses acupuncture, chiropractic, or herbs to manage the disease. And complementary medicine is often high-cost and takes considerable time from the patient's life as he or she visits practitioners more and more.

On the other hand, many complementary providers are also wellness educators at heart; when they set up their practices to spend plenty of time with people, they educate them to understand how they generate their symptoms and how they can have a hand in reducing the frequency of the symptom, thus lowering costs and the frequency of any form of intervention.

When we break the financial conundrum of cost-access-quality by using the continuum model, all sorts of possibilities arise as the medical system is right-sized and used for what it does best, and as the wellness system is used in helping people to live fully and, most importantly, in empowering them to be their own primary-care provider.

Our clinical research over the past 30 years has shown patient satisfaction is NOT correlated with the removal of symptoms; rather, patient satisfaction is most directly correlated with the statement, "I now understand how I control my symptoms." In other words, they are satisfied when they become their own primary care provider.[4]

And that changes the way the cash flows.

NOTES

1. Organisation for Economic Co-operation and Development. *OECD Health Data 2006: Statistics and Indicators for 30 Countries.* See www.oecd.org.

2. Andrew Weil, *Eight Weeks to Optimal Health: A Proven Program for Taking Full Advantage of Your Body's Natural Healing Power* (Ballantine Books, 1998).

3. John Travis and Regina Sara Ryan, *The Wellness Workbook: How to Achieve Enduring Health and Vitality*, 3rd edition (Celestial Arts, 2004).

4. See reports by medical anthropologist Claire Cassidy: "In the Patients' Own Words: Research Report, Part 2," published in *Meridians*, Summer 1997, and "New Research: Patients Vote an Overwhelming 'Yes' for Acupuncture," *Meridians*, Spring 1996.

Part Two: The Opportunity

Grounded Assumptions *for* Health Policy

"Remembering that I'll be dead soon is the most important tool
I've ever encountered to help me make the big choices in life.
Because almost everything – all external expectations, all pride,
all fear of embarrassment or failure – these things just fall away
in the face of death, leaving only what is truly important."[1]
– Steve Jobs

THE QUEST FOR immortality is ageless and exists in all traditions, and usually is understood as eternal life in the spiritual realm after we have left the material realm. In the modern world, however, we are seeing a quest for "eternal life" in the material realm.

As we continue this conversation about health policy in the United States, I suggest it's important to go back to the first essay and review what I have spoken of as highly cherished (and perhaps destructive) certitudes of our modern culture. Briefly, the four assumptions:

- We could find a way to avoid death.

- We could avoid suffering.

- Experts can fix what is called a disease.

- We don't have to take care of ourselves because any illness we generate can be magically corrected by a high-tech intervention.

Those four assumptions drive our modern health-care system. Now it is time for us to look at grounded assumptions based in common sense.

New Assumption: Death as Part of the Cycle of Life

Our current assumption is that we must focus on avoiding death, rather than on bringing peacefulness to each stage of our journey between birth and death. This conversation about death is probably the simplest of the entire book, and also the most difficult. It is at the very heart of the nature of human existence. Depending on how *you* answer this question about death, every other aspect of *your* life is different. Take a moment to reflect on it.

I often say to my patients – people who come to me for assistance, for learning – that when we strip away everything else, the only thing we know for sure is we're here, we were born, and we are going to die. The art of well-living is the art of moving ourselves peacefully between the moment of our birth and the moment of our death. Even with the theoretical possibility of a scientific discovery enabling us to live forever, we cannot live with that supposition today; it is not our current reality. In this time in history, we all will die; and we must design our way of living to recognize that reality and accept death as a part of the natural cycle of life.

" . . . for the past 33 years, I have looked in the mirror every

morning and asked myself: 'If today were the last day of my life, would I want to do what I am about to do today?' And whenever the answer has been 'No' for too many days in a row, I know I need to change something.

"Remembering that I'll be dead soon is the most important tool I've ever encountered to help me make the big choices in life. Because almost everything – all external expectations, all pride, all fear of embarrassment or failure – these things just fall away in the face of death, leaving only what is truly important. Remembering that you are going to die is the best way I know to avoid the trap of thinking you have something to lose. You are already naked. There is no reason not to follow your heart."[1]

– Steve Jobs

If, on the other hand, the purpose is to avoid death at all costs – to prevent and put off death, and to have no suffering between our birth and our death – then an entirely different worldview appears. Ivan Illich, the philosopher, social critic and historian, in 1974 wrote in *Medical Nemesis* (still a major classic) that a culture that sees death as an opponent will begin to spend itself out of existence in trying to conquer it. A culture that accepts death as part of the natural cycle of life will have a very different kind of medicine.[2]

Contrary to popular belief, the per capita cost of health care in Europe and Canada is much lower than in the United States. No nation on the planet comes close to the US in cost per capita or cost as a percentage of GDP. It may be that this difference in cost is more closely related to a different attitude about death and suffering than to anything else. The lower costs elsewhere may result from the greater acceptance within those cultures of the nature of life as a progression between birth and death.[3]

To my knowledge, all of the great world traditions, unlike those of the modern West, accept that the cause of suffering in life is the expectation that life be different than exactly how it is. Thus when we set up an expectation, e.g., "My spouse will begin to behave differently than she/he has in the past 20 years," we set ourselves up for pain. Americans are at a crossroads: Are humans able to overcome the nature of life as it is? Or must we learn to live with the laws of nature and with life as it is? For much of the Industrial Age, the West has seen itself as powerful enough to overcome storms, cyclones, hurricanes, fires, and tornadoes. In recent years, however, we've become aware that perhaps we can't conquer all of nature.

Perhaps we must shift that conversation and realize, as the environmental movement has taught us, that we are part of the system of nature and we had best learn to live with it rather than pretend humans can overcome it.

This is the basic philosophical conversation. Are we humans in charge of nature, or are we part of the cycle of nature? Are humans a part of tending the cycle of life, or are we able to dominate the cycle of life? Clearly, much of the scientific activity and efforts of the twentieth century were dedicated to the assumption that humans could create utopia without having to deal with pain, suffering, and death.

In my clinical experience, I've been at the bedside of someone who was dying, along with the person's wonderful physician. The doctor said, "For me, this is a moment of failure." And then, looking over at me, the doctor continued: "For you, this is a moment of success. I have failed because I have not prevented death. You have been successful because you have taught this person the art of dying peacefully."

So, dear reader, you must ask yourself the question, "Am I ready to accept death as part of the cycle of life?" In the first essay we spoke of Larry and Peg, of Larry's peaceful transition, and the money saved by a decision they made about this question at Johns Hopkins Hospital.

My fourth-grade teacher introduced the fact of death as a part of life when she said as we were leaving class each day, "Now, before you go to bed tonight, are you at peace with everyone you love and everyone in your family? You don't know who will not wake up in the morning." I often think that Sister Jean Marie, who asked that question every day and coached us nine year olds to be loving and peaceful and forgiving, now would likely be sued or banished from teaching for raising the issue of death with youngsters. It probably would be considered abusive. However, death – how we think about and deal with death – is a core issue.

I was asked one day to tend a bishop who was suffering with cancer. He was a man near 70, and his friends wanted me to tend him so he would be restored to full functioning and recover from cancer. When I met him, I asked the question, "You've been telling all of us for many years to behave so that we would be welcomed into heaven. You now have a straight, quick shot at heaven. The Lord has delivered this mystery called cancer to you. I don't understand why you're fighting it with chemotherapy. Why are you in resistance to the natural course of life?" He hadn't been asked this question before. No one had ever raised the question with him that he frequently raised from the pulpit: What is the purpose of life? What is the meaning of the moment of death? How do we die with glory? I asked the bishop, "Is there anything you have to do before you let go?" "Oh, yes, there are these two projects." "Well, are you going to do them?" "Oh, yes," he said.

The next day, the bishop apparently had a remarkable recovery. He completed both of those projects over the next several months. Then, to everyone's astonishment, he very quickly passed away. A problem? Or a glorious, full living of life?

Another New Assumption: Life is Difficult, and Suffering is Part of Life

We assume life should be without suffering; and we know by experience this assumption is false. Scott Peck's bestselling book, *The Road Less Traveled,* begins with these words: "Life is difficult." Yet our health-care system is predicated on an assumption that we can prevent life's difficulties, resulting in an endless attempt to find the drug or the surgery that will remove all suffering. This philosophy of doing away with suffering coincides with many other assumptions about life, such as the idea we can control ecosystems and avoid damage from floods, fires, or hurricanes. What we have here is a philosophy that humans can control nature – a philosophy we are beginning to realize is deeply mistaken. (I repeat all this because until we acknowledge this reality and deal with it appropriately, we will continue to harm our people and bankrupt our nation.)

In expense terms, we have made the avoidance of suffering a trillion-dollar industry by means of drugs, medications, plastic surgery, and many other therapies. The question of how we deal with the triangle of cost-quality-access must start with a decision about our values. Are we designing our life (our way of being in life as a community, a culture) as a way of helping each other to move peacefully from our birth through a life that includes suffering and learning how to deal with life's suffering?

I think of John Weadock's fullness of life as he lived without complaint for 40 years in a wheelchair. (See Essay 1.)

The following pages are predicated on the crazy assumption that the real issue in the modern world is "How do you move with relative ease and peacefulness between the time of birth and the time of death?" *I suggest that the effort to be "healthy" is a modern addiction that prevents us from learning the art of living so that we can move with ease from day to day.*

If you go running today for the pleasure it brings, for the

freedom you feel as the wind passes by you, that is one thing. However, if you are forcing yourself to get up and run today so you won't die prematurely 30 years from now, that's very different and is an out-of-the-present-moment body experience.

Before you read the next pages, be sure you have come to some internal clarity about your own value decisions concerning the issues surrounding death and suffering; and realize that if you are choosing prevention of death and prevention of suffering, you are making an economically irrational choice. As a modern Western culture, we've been making that choice for about 50 years with virtually zero success. No doctor has prevented death; no doctor has prevented suffering. At best, doctors have prolonged life and alleviated suffering. And we know many of the interventions to prevent suffering seem to have unexpected side consequences which, perhaps, make life's suffering even more complicated.

So be sure you have answered the question for yourself: Are you learning the art of living, including living with the sufferings of life – physical, emotional, and social – and how to bear with suffering and create ease with suffering? Or are you in a game of attempting to prevent suffering and death? Both choices have enormous economic consequences for you, for your family, for your grandchildren, and for our entire society.

Assumption: Tend the *Whole* Person

If we choose to be in a fight with life, we also assume there are experts who can fix the disease we bring to them. William Osler, considered the founder of modern medicine, often said, "It is much more important to know what sort of patient has a disease than what sort of disease the patient has."[4]

I have a personal story that illustrates what can happen when the practitioner focuses on the disease and not the whole person. It happened the first time a physician referred a patient to me because he was afraid that drug interactions were affecting his patient, the result of having referred her to five different specialists for five different diseases. The woman was being seen by a pulmonologist for her asthma, a urologist for urinary tract infections and lack of control, a gastroenterologist for irritable bowel symptoms, a gynecologist for irregular and painful periods, and an orthopedic physician for back pain. Each specialist had prescribed medications, and her primary care physician was now concerned the interactions among the five drugs were creating more problems than the original diseases. Each specialist was looking at his or her own piece of the puzzle. The woman had brought her symptom – the breathing problem, the urinary problem, etc. – and asked the specialist to fix that particular part. Here we have the modern woman with the modern specialists, each specialist in a war with his/her particular disease, no one seeing the whole, and more tragically, no one even knowing how to see the whole. Soon after taking a different perspective focused on lifestyle changes, this woman no longer needed medical specialists.

I empathize with medical specialists who tend parts of a human and have never learned the joy of tending a whole person. To me, it is amazing even to consider that one human can tend another human being as a collection of parts without being aware that this isn't how his/her own body works.

Modern patients have been trained to present a ticket, a particular symptom that they feel is a valid reason for seeking care. Our medical system then codes that symptom for insurance reimbursement. The practitioner gets paid for piecemeal work – for applying techniques to a particular diseased part of the individual, usually with the implicit assumption that it is self-contained.

We're going to see the impact of the whole-person approach in the next essay where we look at existing communities that do not focus on specialization or the individual's "ticket," but on the wholeness of the human organism, with each symptom reflecting the holography of the unique individual.

Assumption: Our Mind and Body Are Totally Interactive

We also live as if our mind is not connected to our body. We assume the body does what it does; and somehow, magically, our mind, our way of living, our attitudes are not connected to the well-being of our body. This is an assumption that comes from 400 years of thinking of the mind and body as separate realities. As neuroscientist Candace Pert pointed out in her 1993 PBS interview with Bill Moyers, the separation of the mind and the body was a deal between Descartes and the Pope, in which the Pope got to control the mind and the spirit, and the body was left to Descartes and to other physical scientists who followed. People gradually began to turn to experts to fix their body because they assumed their attitudes and ways of living had nothing to do with their body's symptoms.[5]

I've been thinking a lot about what we call the obesity epidemic in the United States, specifically of a family I've known for more than 40 years. When I first met them, all of the family members – the elders and the young ones – were slender and energetic; they knew how to support themselves from the land; they were active and out in the world. Forty years later, no one in the group hunts or grows food any longer; they buy everything from the store, and they are all obese. Now they eat mainly packaged, chemicalized foods and have no sense of why they are obese. All of them are on many medications and drugs. They no longer know their body. They're not in charge of their body. They're not in charge of their life. Everything is turned over to "Well, my doctor says . . . "

This "turn it over to the doctor/specialist" attitude encourages daily behavior that assumes the human can live however he or she wants without regard for the impact it has on health and wellness.

This Is Common Sense

There is a nationwide movement to change these attitudes and re-gain control of our health care. However, many things impede the change, including: (1) the existing policies of the medical monopo-ly, pharmaceutical monopoly, and food monopoly; and (2) the dan-gerous modern cultural assumptions that we mindlessly pass on to our children. These personal and corporate assumptions require mindful reexamination. Awakening to a new set of assumptions will bring huge financial benefits plus greater dignity to the quality of life in American society.

These more realistic assumptions – assumptions that have us deal with life as it actually shows up – enable a radical transforma-tion of the way we think about wellness, health, the health-care system, and health-care financing. These clearer assumptions en-able us to break the iron triangle of health care – cost, access, qual-ity – and create new possibilities.

NOTES

1. Steve Jobs, in his commencement address at Stanford University, June 12, 2005. Available at news.stanford.edu/news/2005/june15/jobs-061505.

2. See Ivan Illich, *Limits to Medicine: Medical Nemesis, the Expropriation of Health*. (London, England: Marion Boyars Publishers, Ltd., 2000).

3. Daniel Callahan, "Health Care Costs and Medical Technology," in *From Birth to Death and Bench to Clinic: The Hastings Center Bioethics Briefing Book for Journalists, Policymakers, and Campaigns*, ed. Mary Crowley (Garrison, NY: The Hastings Center, 2008), 79-82.

4. This quote from Osler is based on the words of Hippocrates, often called the father of Western medicine, who lived in the fifth and fourth centu-ries, BC. His influential writings, including the Hippocratic Oath, are collected in *The Corpus: The Hippocratic Writings (Kaplan Classics of Medicine)*. Kaplan Publishing, original edition, 2008.

5. Candace Pert, PhD, was one of the scientific experts interviewed in Bill Moyers' highly acclaimed 1993 PBS series, Healing and the Mind.

New Assumptions – Thriving Communities

"Traditionally, medical care has focused on treating and curing disease. We need to focus more on keeping people healthy."
– Delos M. Cosgrove, MD, President and CEO, Cleveland Clinic Health System

Pay your physician to keep you well,
and the physician pays the patients if they get sick.
– Chinese Proverb

I HAVE ASSERTED a set of new assumptions on which to base our health care – assumptions that may enable us to enrich our wellness and our social systems. Although these assumptions may *seem* new, they are deeply-rooted, core American values. They are rooted in the empowerment of individuals, the awakening of a mindful presence to the bodily senses and how individuals live well and fully. By *mindful presence,* I mean the kind of full attention we bring to sports or dancing or cooking or our love of being in nature.

Mindful awakening of the senses puts the individual and the

family at the core of their own well-being, reducing their dependence on experts and, essentially, having individuals and family communities become their own primary care provider. They become their own provider by increasing awareness of the way their body and emotions are affected by the way they eat, the way they move and exercise, and by the way they speak with friends and family.

Naturally, the question arises as to whether there is any evidence that our new assumptions are viable in the practical day-to-day world of modern America. Happily, we find many successful demonstration projects, educational programs, and initiatives already in place to show such a way of living is not only possible but financially viable – and there is extensive academic research from very credible sources pointing to this approach as an essential way forward.

These assumptions are deeply rooted in the background of our society and culture at every level. As of yet, however, they are not thought of as a way to build an innovative new approach in which funding shifts from dependence on experts to reliance on enhanced awareness and enriched styles of living.

These assumptions are not based on the prevention of disease; they are based on the art of successful living. Our nation's first lady, Michele Obama, has been promoting exercise, healthy food, and the gardening of organic food at the White House. However, what she is doing often is presented in terms of preventing disease and preventing obesity. There are many fun photos showing the Obama children and local school children working in the White House garden, planting and harvesting food. Those photos resonate with all of us. What if we shifted from speaking about preventing disease toward a focus on the joy of gardening and eating and cooking healthy foods because *you feel better right now*? You are enjoying life; you are experiencing nature; you are experiencing the connection with food and air – and it has an immediate present-moment payoff. You feel empowered. You are not dependent on experts to grow and deliver your food.

Same activities, different speaking, deeper speaking. And with deeper speaking, I suggest a deeper resonance, a deeper acceptance of life, a deeper wisdom about living well.

Substantial evidence shows that individuals who understand how their body works have a different level of life satisfaction than those for whom the body is a mystery tended by professional health-care providers. Two examples:

I knew a second-year medical student at the University of Pennsylvania Medical School who was about to have throat surgery for a painful lump in his throat. Both his internist and the surgeon agreed that the only way to deal with this growth was to undergo surgery. When he was led through a series of body self-awareness exercises, he began to cry over the amount of stress in his life – and the lump went away overnight. He had been unaware that his throat tightened whenever he was *"stressed,"* and that this tightness was a sign of excess tension in his life. When he broke the tension, the painful obstruction went away. Throat surgery or self-awareness? This young man was about to go out into the world as a medical student, unaware of the useful signs within his body for guiding him in living well. Our student had never been taught to be an observer of his own body.

Another example is a 35-year-old former professional athlete, Gary, the father of two young children, who now works in our national security system. Gary lost a large clump of hair and saw his physician, who began to treat him for the diagnosis, alopecia (hair loss). A few weeks later, Gary had back pain and was treated with a muscle relaxant and pain relievers. A month after that, he had a urinary tract infection and saw another physician, who gave him another medication. None of the physicians asked him about sleep or rest, about stress or anxiety. Gary routinely gets about six hours of sleep; he often works at night as part of his Homeland Security job and considers himself highly "stressed" and exhausted. He now has seen three physicians who, based on their training, have correctly diagnosed his condition as several individual diseases and have tended those diseases without any attempt to promote overall wellness, or even awareness.

I have practiced healing medicine for 40 years from a different perspective, and I see all of his symptoms as physical manifestations of exhaustion, stress, and anxiety. Yet throughout his treatment, these symptoms were not tended or even mentioned by his doctors.

As expressed by the CEO of the Cleveland Clinic, Delos Cosgrove, MD, we have a disease-care system, not a wellness system. We're focused on fighting disease and preventing disease. We do not have a focus on living fully. Significant evidence indicates that more than 75 percent of visits to medical offices are for chronic functional disorders – ways in which our bodies are not working well and should be treated by lifestyle changes.[1]

What if the essential outcome for change in our health-care system is an enhanced self-awareness of how our own body works, of how our mind and body are coordinated, of how our body guides, signals, and alerts us to make changes. In the present system, a six-year-old is diagnosed with ADHD and prescribed a drug he will take for many years. Alternatively, this first grader could be taught yoga and breathing exercises. Evidence shows that breathing, yoga, and relaxation techniques in the classroom link to higher learning scores and more focused students. More importantly, perhaps, our six-year-old learns to breathe, stretch, exercise, and manage his body, enjoying the benefits of these practices throughout a lifetime – and it's free.

If given a prescription drug, the child learns that the way you manage your body is by going to an expert who delivers a chemical – and it's expensive. If taught to breathe and stretch, the child learns that wellness is part of our birthright and can be learned. We have the choice.

Empowerment is a common thread. A few years ago, I led a workshop at the Schumacher College in Devon, England. One of the participants was a woman who worked at a cancer care centre in Bristol, England, a clinic known for being among the most cutting-edge over the past 30 years in finding innovative ways to help people who have been labeled with cancer. The woman announced that after many years of working at the centre, she was leaving to found a new clinic nearby. While she had not yet formulated a name for the new clinic, she said the name that goes on the door should carry this message: "You don't have to get cancer in order to wake up and learn how to live fully." Her goal was to teach people to live fully and to maximize their life experience. Taking this approach to life can change the course of any disease.

I am not naïve, although many may think so. I am well aware that I am taking the long view, a generational view. This is not about change within the next financial reporting period or in the term of one president. We have taken 100 years to create our almost total dependence on experts, generating the extreme financial and social difficulties in which we now find ourselves as a nation. It may take some time to shift the direction back to the empowerment of the individual and change society's relationship with experts to an appropriate one. And now is the time.

At this moment there are many financial and social forces aligned to make a significant start for the sake of our next generations, of our children and grandchildren. Many well-designed programs are demonstrating the value of empowering individuals to maximize their own wellness. Here are several examples:

Programs that Empower Individuals

The Cleveland Clinic Employee Wellness Program (www.cchs. net/wellness). In a document published in 2006, Delos Cosgrove, MD, President and CEO of the Cleveland Clinic Health System, observes:

"Traditionally, medical care has focused on treating and curing disease. Today, we are starting to focus on wellness; and we're beginning with our own employees. There is compelling evidence to support that healthy employees have lower medical costs and higher productivity. For these reasons, we are creating an innovative, high-quality employee wellness program."[2]

This was a major event. Wellness used to be relegated to a particular New Age demographic that frequented the strange health-food store in the neighborhood. Now, wellness and resources for wellness such as the Cleveland Clinic program are a mainstream necessity. The Clinic employs 34,000 individuals, and that means shifting the expenditure of many millions of health-care dollars from disease care to preventing disease by promoting well-living.

We must acknowledge the internal conflict of financial interests highlighted by this event. The more that Clinic employees make use of the medical services, the more money the insurance provider pays the Clinic. The more that Clinic employees make use of the wellness programs, the fewer hospital admissions, i.e., loss of business. However, since the Cleveland Clinic is self-insured, the less employees use the medical system, the more money is saved by the Clinic.[3]

Several hospital presidents have said to me (off the record, of course): "Bob, I can't afford to get people well. I wake up praying for more surgery patients so that we can pay the bills." Dr. Cosgrove must be commended for his courage in taking his high-minded stance.

This program is focused on wellness as a means of preventing disease and on managing the behavior of individuals toward long-term goals. However, it is also an educational program that empowers individuals, bringing awareness of their bodies and control of their daily lives. It will have a long-term impact as individuals learn that stress and upset are optional and are changed by breathing, sleep, exercise, and good food habits.

For companies that manufacture widgets or legal documents, or for schools that teach the next generations of our youth, such a program brings no conflict of interest. Applying similar program principles is a business decision that benefits both employees and the financial bottom line.

Dow Chemical's Wellness Initiative (www.dow.com/familyhealth/health). Dow Chemical may be well ahead of the Cleveland Clinic. An international conglomerate with over 50,000 employees world-wide, Dow Chemical has invested heavily in wellness program-ming for all of its employees in recent years. Dow's Global Director of Health Services, Catherine Baase, MD, testified before the US Senate Committee on Health, Education, Labor and Pensions in February 2009, reporting that for companies with comprehen-sive health promotion programs, studies indicated a return of at least three dollars in costs saved for every dollar spent on wellness. Nearly ten years ago, Dow's business case analysis indicated that by keeping their inflation rates for health-care expenses at a best performance level – similar to consumer price inflation rather than the much higher rate of medical inflation – they could potentially save $420 million over ten years and up to ten cents per share by 2013. In fact, they have tracked their actual savings and noted that between a baseline year of 2004 and 2011 they saved at least $120 million. Dr. Baase indicated wellness programs were a key part of their efforts, which enabled the corporation to stabilize the rate of increase in medical health-care expenses to an average of two per-cent for the previous five years. (This during a time when general health-care inflation was in the range of eight to nine percent per year.)

Imagine the total contribution to Dow Chemical's bottom line from such savings. Imagine their corporate competitive advantage in the marketplace. Imagine applying this trajectory of savings to the 50 billion dollars spent annually by the US military on the medical and health-related expenses of their troops and families and civilian employees. Imagine the impact on our federal budget of applying these principles to all Medicare recipients and to all the employees in the federal workforce. We are talking big dollars saved using well-demonstrated approaches.

Researchers may argue about the double-blind evidence for the effectiveness of specific wellness initiatives; however there is no arguing about the outcomes data such as that shown by Dow Chemical and many similar corporate initiatives.

InspireHealth (www.inspirehealth.ca). The government of the Canadian Province of British Columbia recently funded the expansion of a program called InspireHealth, located in Vancouver. InspireHealth has served individuals with cancer since 1997. Research indicates that individuals with a serious cancer diagnosis who fully participate in this integrative care program improved outcomes compared to patients who have access only to the conventional system. The patients at InspireHealth have available all of the surgical, chemotherapy and radiation options provided in the conventional system; however, as they begin this normal course of treatment for cancer, they also begin a learning process about the foundations of health. They are guided by coaches in the use of food, herbs, movement, breathing, yoga, acupuncture, and other forms of care that maximize well-being and enhance the immune system.

The program begins with the most basic ideas about wellness, as reflected in this pyramid illustration of the most basic elements essential for wellness. For patients to experience the maximum benefits of radiation, chemotherapy and surgery, wellness practices are held as essential. These practices include a healthful diet, plenty of sleep and rest, relaxation, appropriate exercise, and the development of skills for emotional wellness and body-mind awareness.[4]

The program teaches the same basic skills of wellness to an

InspireHealth Foundations of Health and Healing

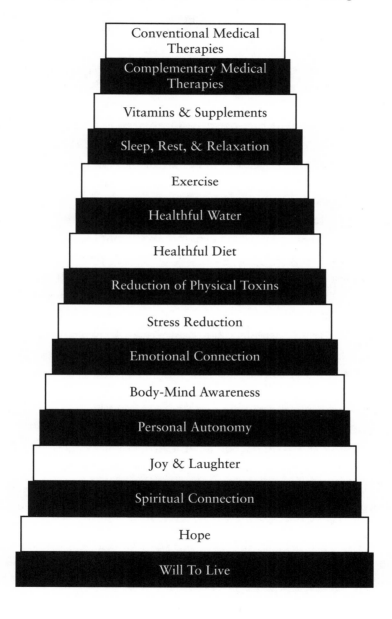

Conventional Medical Therapies

Complementary Medical Therapies

Vitamins & Supplements

Sleep, Rest, & Relaxation

Exercise

Healthful Water

Healthful Diet

Reduction of Physical Toxins

Stress Reduction

Emotional Connection

Body-Mind Awareness

Personal Autonomy

Joy & Laughter

Spiritual Connection

Hope

Will To Live

individual who has been diagnosed with a serious illness as should be taught to all of us in society as part of life.

Although this program starts with individuals who have been diagnosed with a serious illness, the core of the program is about teaching everyone – those who are ill as well as those without a diagnosis – how to live well. The program is applicable to everyone, and thus is shared with family and friends and becomes a way of living.

The government of British Columbia recently allocated funding for expansion of this Vancouver program; and it allocated 2.5 million Canadian dollars annually to bring this program to four other sites in British Columbia, making it available to many more people. The evidence suggests that the program promotes improved quality of life and longevity, brings exceptional patient satisfaction, and has better outcomes than conventional approaches. The Samueli Institute, a US-based research organization with a focus on healing, has identified InspireHealth as a leading example of an optimal healing environment, and has received a $2 million grant to further the benefits of InspireHealth's programs. Those outcomes are clearly demonstrated. What also should be clear is that when people are living healthier lives and living longer without disease, they are more productive members of society and are costing the health-care system less.

This is not to say education about healthy practices alone will prevent disease. Such learning, however, maximizes people's awareness about living well, whether or not they have a disease; and if a disease does manifest, they are better prepared to cope with it. What would the outcomes be if people had all these skills for healthy living before they had to cope with the mystery we label "cancer"?

The Culm Valley Health Centre (www.culmvalleynaturalhealth. co.uk). Based in Cullompton, Devon, England, the Culm Valley

experiment is a relatively small project devised to provide treatment for those relatively few individuals in a very wealthy county who do not have access to health insurance. Normally, such individuals get care only when their need is complicated and they are forced to go to the emergency room; they get care only when what might have been a symptom (and could have been tended routinely) has become an expensive pathology.

Healthy Howard is set up to provide care for individuals as needed, regardless of insurance. The premise of the care is that each person who participates must be involved in learning about his/her own wellness through regularly scheduled meetings with a health coach, with whom they review their health status and life activities around food, exercise, and all the aspects of life that maximize well living.

This program is conducted in collaboration with the County Health Department and the Howard County General Hospital, which is part of the Johns Hopkins Medical System. The project is also reviewed by researchers from the Johns Hopkins School of Public Health. The early outcomes from this program indicate that those who are engaged with health coaches have a lower incidence of admission to the emergency room and require fewer hospital admissions in general. Thus the core of the program – up-front coaching in the basics of maintaining well-being, combined with a primary-care medical home – has a financial benefit in reduced hospital admissions. This program has been cited by Senator Barbara Mikulski in formal US Senate hearings held both on Capitol Hill and at the Health Department in Howard County. She has pointed to Healthy Howard as an example of the value of wellness promotion before onset of disease, and as an approach that can have a major impact on health-care costs in America.

Maryland Community Health Initiative, "Penn North" (www. penn-north.org), is a program that I have been deeply involved in developing over the past 15 years and is currently directed by my son, Blaize Connelly-Duggan. Penn North is located near the corner of Pennsylvania and North Avenues in Baltimore, an area at the center of much crime and poverty. The program serves more than 350 people each day in a small, 3,000-square-foot space. Most participants are in recovery from the use of cocaine, heroin, and other street drugs, and many of them have spent time in jail for drug-related events. Many also have serious medical and mental-health diagnoses. They are a population costing the health-care and the criminal justice systems enormous funds. More than 7,000 unique individuals make use of Penn North services every year.

One of the initial directors of Penn North, Al Duha Chase, a man who had spent considerable time in prison and who later trained as a tai chi master, spoke of the work of Penn North in this way: *"As a street person in Baltimore, heroin was for me a very faithful friend. If you want me off my heroin, you had better build me a friendship community."* That's the core idea of Penn North: provide a place where people can gather day or night (the space is open from 8 a.m. to 2 a.m.), so when there is an urge to use a drug, a person can visit the Penn North community for support. Support appears in many ways – it might be participating in a Narcotics Anonymous meeting, playing a domino game, doing tai chi or yoga, working on a high-school equivalency diploma, learning computer skills, participating in the job readiness program, having an acupuncture treatment, or receiving long-term intensive counseling. This is all part of an entire package of support that begins when the person comes through Penn North's door and is greeted by Donnetta, Natalie, Ben, or Vernard, who for more than ten years have been our community outreach workers, the creators of a convivial family atmosphere. This support continues with the nurturing attention of all the other individuals who use the small space. That caring community generates a "stickiness," a long-term participation in the community itself as a basic life support.

An early study as well as anecdotal reports point to a significant reduction in participants' return to prison; however, funding has not been available to closely measure outcomes, including findings of reduced prison recidivism and lowered admissions to emergency rooms.

A very low-cost program (approximately $6 per individual visit), Penn North illustrates how a low-budget community-level initiative can lower hospital admissions and prevent returns to prison simply by the availability of an alternative community and a place to learn skills for living well.

Alcoholics Anonymous (www.aa.org), with its ubiquitous meetings and its simple twelve steps to self-awareness and self-responsibility, is perhaps the largest worldwide demonstration of the concept we are discussing. Imagine the added expense to our health-care system if there were no such support system for those who have become non-functional as a result of alcohol. AA is a system that builds relationships among people, essentially a place where they teach each other how to live well in line with the twelve steps, the basic rules for living life. As such principles are applied widely, not just as a response to disease but as principles for living, and as communities cultivate groups to better understand life well lived, I believe health-care costs will decline just as costs are controlled when individuals participate in AA.

All of these examples have common threads. These examples do not start from the assumption that life is a fight with death and disease requiring dependence on high-tech experts; they start with the assumption that our bodies are inherently wise and individuals are capable of self-healing except in limited, unusual circumstances.

Each program revolves around the empowerment of the individual, around self-care in which individuals learn how their body works and how to care for themselves. People recover simple knowledge about how to intervene early in simple ways when a symptom shows up. These programs engage the power of personal mindfulness; they generate awareness; they are rooted in teaching basic life practices such as movement, breathing, and eating well; they are based on community.

The extraordinary outcomes result from a real-time, pleasant, and full participation in life. None of these outcomes results from a focus on fighting a disease, although the reduced occurrence and severity of disease is a by-product. All of these examples involve low-tech, low-cost activities that discourage reliance on more costly high-tech resources. All of the outcomes point to the value of an enhanced sense of well-being in real time.

These are seven illustrations. There are hundreds of such initiatives. They are not well linked. They are not framed as potential components of a larger national policy. They are initiatives created out of locally perceived need and benefit – local initiatives with enormous potential for national impact. They point to ways our nation can start shifting the expenditure of $1.2 trillion from a fight with disease into the promotion of happiness, wellness, and empowerment through right living.

Widely Available Instructional Resources

In addition to such projects there are deep instructional resources, available online and in other media, which provide the simple resources the public needs to refocus on wellness. A few examples:

The Blue Zones. An ABC *20/20* report titled "Secrets of Happiness – Blue Zones" tells the story of four places in the world where a remarkable number of people live into their nineties and beyond. It was based on *The Blue Zones,* a widely-read bestseller by Dan Buettner, who had travelled the planet to find the world's longest-lived people and explore their lifestyles. Buettner subsequently discovered additional Blue Zones, including the Greek island of Ikaria, where a monk was filmed giving a tour. We see the monk, who is in his nineties, riding along on his motorbike and stopping on the roadside to pick plants, herbs, and berries, which he describes as a wonderful part of the Ikarians' diet. The monk attributes their longevity to the qualities of the foods they eat.[5,6]

Another Blue Zone is in Southern California, in the Loma Linda area, where there is an unusually high rate of longevity. Loma Linda is a major center of the Adventist Church, which focuses on vegetarian food and good lifestyles. In the 1800s and early 1900s, a spa/sanitarium based on health principles advocated by the Adventist Church was an important part of an American movement toward healthy eating and healthy living. The superintendent of that health resort and his brother were inspired by these wellness principles and applied them when they moved on to found the Kellogg Company and create the Kellogg Foundation. As we enter the twenty-first century, the healthy eating and healthy living encouraged in Blue Zones such as Loma Linda potentially may serve as a great way of living life for most of the world's population.

Our national goal must be to bring into the mainstream ways of living well that are practiced in Loma Linda and the other rare zones on our planet. The mainstream ways of living recovered in Loma Linda are reminders of what is possible.

In these Blue Zones we have a living knowledge resource about how to live well, derived from cultures where people live longer and better with very little medicalization, very little hospitalization, very little interference in the natural course of life. If you listen carefully to the people in these zones, they are saying much of what we have pointed to in these essays: *Living well is common sense.*

This example of the Blue Zones emphasizes what we all recognize as well-living, such as having purpose, appropriate rest, appropriate food, fun, family, a sense of belonging, and concern for the well-being of the tribe. These ways of wellness are common sense and well documented; they are not "New Age" – they are at the bedrock of American values.

Influential leaders, books, television programs, and Senate hearings. As a further example of the widespread movement focusing on wellness in our nation, I point to Andrew Weil's *Eight Weeks to Optimal Health*, first published in 1997. Dr. Weil describes the basics of what it means to live well. He speaks of food, of sleep, of what we drink and natural products; he also describes taking a "news fast" and learning how to meditate and create inner peace. At a 2009 Senate hearing, Dr. Weil mentioned such ways of maximizing the body's innate ability to stay healthy.

In 1997, James Gordon, MD, published *Manifesto for a New Medicine*. He later served as Chair of the White House Commission on Complementary Medicine, and founded the Center for Mind-Body Medicine in Washington, DC. The Center now teaches self-care in Israel, Gaza, Haiti, Kosovo, and New Orleans, as well as in the Washington, DC, area.

Dr. Gordon and Dr. Weil are reflective of a large movement which includes, for example, the work of Dean Ornish on heart disease, the commonsense advice of Mehmet Oz in his television presentations and appearances with Oprah Winfrey, and the work of physician John Travis, who opened the first wellness center in 1975 and whose books include *The Wellness Workbook*.

Deepak Chopra and David Simon have made extensive contributions to the wellness movement, including books they co-authored where, based on their medical background, they point to what happens in medicine when we ignore the mind and the spirit and neglect our relationship with nature.[7]

US Senate Committee Hearings in February 2009 focused on wellness as an effective path for our nation and provided a wide outline of practical resources and wisdom. (Hearings of the US

Senate Committee on Health, Education, Labor, and Pensions are available online at www.help.senate.gov.)

The work of Martin Seligman, PhD, in establishing the field now called "positive psychology." His most recent book, *Flourish,* is about human beings learning to live a fulfilling and joyful life as opposed to becoming caught up in a disease model.[8]

Dr. Seligman's work, similar to that of Dr. Weil and his colleagues, focuses research on what generates happiness and optimism. A professor of psychology at the University of Pennsylvania, he looks into what happens when people are living well and the characteristics and practices that enable a good life. This approach is very distinct from the research at the university's medical school.

In "Army Strong," chapter six of *Flourish,* Dr. Seligman reports on his collaboration with the US Army in its desire to enable wellness and resilience at all levels of military life, from combat duties to family time. The entire military community must flourish if the mission is to be achieved.

Dr. Seligman is one example of many available resources on how to generate happiness – a conversation distinct from research on how individuals fight illness. I think of John Haidt's work at the University of Virginia and his book, *The Happiness Hypothesis.*[9] Many more examples are cited in the November/December 2011 issue of *Resurgence.* (www.resurgence.org)

The Search Institute in Minneapolis, Minnesota (www.search-institute.org), while focused specifically on promoting success at the elementary and high school levels of education, points to basic life habits for success in education similar to those essential for success in wellness. Since the 1980s, the Search Institute has looked at the qualities of students who do well in grade school and high school. They have identified and researched 40 positive qualities (20 inner and 20 outer traits, practices, and habits of being) that point toward a person's ability to be highly functional in our society. Teachers love this approach because, when dealing with a student, it shifts the focus from the problem-base to the asset-base.

These 40 assets are very simple: dinner with family several times a week, having elders in their lives outside the immediate family, ability to spend time alone, being curious about reading, etc. These seemingly simple traits are the basis for success.

In summary, the qualities we point to here resonate with the work of Andy Weil, with what is taken for granted in the Blue Zones, and what Marty Seligman is talking about in *Flourish*. They also are qualities we honor in special military groups such as the Navy SEALs, who have honed the body, mind, and spirit as one. We glorify these groups without stopping to think that we can apply their wellness philosophies in the world of health care. We do the same with many aspects of sports and the arts – glorify and don't stop to think of the possibilities for daily life.

This knowledge is available through a variety of sources, including resources noted in this essay. We've seen this approach applied with excellent results on the football field, the battlefield, and in communities across the world that have not lost their wellness traditions. While the medical industry and politicians haven't necessarily gotten the message, individuals the world over are awakening to the common sense that it is time to make a bridge from the world of disease to new practices that enable quality of living.

Academic Resources

Finally, we point to academic resources. It's often asked, "But where is the research to support these ideas and practices?" The simple answer is that there is abundant research; and because it does not flow from our cherished and accepted (and I say destructive) assumptions, we are on "automatic" to ignore this extensive body of knowledge that has often been paid for by taxpayer funds.

The Samueli Institute in Alexandria, Virginia (www.samueliinstitute.org). The Samueli Institute was a major impetus for me to write this book. During a visit to the Institute I walked through a long hallway where the walls were lined with research documenting the scientific basis for wellness in America. I was overwhelmed as I realized the extent of the solid outcomes data about healing and wellness practices, and at the same time realized how few of these well-documented practices are part of daily life in American families and communities, and how seldom they are discussed in the media.

The Samueli Institute was conceived by Wayne Jonas, MD, with the collaboration of Henry and Susan Samueli. Dr. Jonas, former US Army physician and National Institutes of Health (NIH) researcher, heads the Samueli Institute based in Alexandria, Virginia, and Newport Beach, California. Since 2001, Samueli has been gathering, conducting and funding research on optimal healing environments and practices, whole-person health promotion systems, and community wellness and resilience programs – putting the science behind how people heal and can become and remain well. They have a vast set of academic resources and information, which they apply in collaboration with a number of groups including the US Military, the Veterans Administration, hospitals, worksites, and community organizations. They are leading the Wellness Initiative for the Nation (WIN), described in a summary document in the Appendix. WIN paints a compelling vision of how national policy, along with industry and community leaders, can create a flourishing society for our children and our future.

In addition to his role as President and CEO of the Samueli Institute, Dr. Jonas is an Associate Professor of Family Medicine at the Uniformed Services University of Health Sciences. He served as a military doctor and is now a retired US Army Lieutenant Colonel. He was Director of the Medical Research Fellowship at the Walter Reed Army Institute, a member of the White House Commission on Complementary and Alternative Medicine Policy, and from 1995 to 1999 was Director of the Office of Alternative Medicine at the National Institutes of Health. He also is a sensitive healer who brings this range of experience to his leadership of Samueli. I cite these credentials because they indicate that a man of considerable experience stands behind the work of this Institute.

In collaboration with the Samueli Institute, the Bravewell Collaborative and other groups, the Institute of Medicine convened the "Summit on Integrative Medicine and the Health of the Public" in February 2009. The Summit issued a report strongly endorsing the tools available for promoting wellness and for shifting America from a disease model to a wellness model. Subsequently, several organizations, including the American Association of Retired Persons (AARP), joined in a project that supports this approach to health care with ongoing activities.[10]

The research writings of Nortin Hadler, MD, a professor at the University of North Carolina, who has studied and written extensively about the pitfalls of our medical system. In *The Last Well Person* and *Worried Sick,* he points to the victimization that occurs when individuals lose awareness of their ability to maintain their life skills through exercise, diet, and a limited, appropriate use of experts. In *The Last Well Person,* Dr. Hadler remarks that one of the most dangerous things a person can do before age 85 is to allow himself/herself to be diagnosed by a physician or by anyone else. In other words, it is dangerous for individuals to turn over awareness of their own wellness status to another person.[11]

Resources emphasizing the importance of the whole-person perspective. Abraham Verghese, MD, professor at Stanford University

School of Medicine, points to the lack of a skill-set among physicians that enables them to fully know and engage with the patient and to be in the presence of the whole person – not "specializing," but understanding the patient's entire life circumstance, history, and attitude, and how they interplay with many distinct symptoms all at once.[12] Similarly, Atul Gawande, MD, in his *New Yorker* article, "The Hot Spotters," notes the loss of this holistic perspective in the world of specialists, a perspective that enables significant cost-cutting in the medical health-care system.[13]

There is a vast literature on wellness at the practical, theoretical, and academic levels. Please see the extensive citations in the WIN (Wellness Initiative for the Nation) document in the appendix.

Conclusion

Americans must build a bridge from the world of disease to the world of wellness. It is time to bring this knowledge forward and put it in place through wellness teachers functioning in many settings across our nation.

A popular reality show, "The Biggest Loser," is designed around extremely obese people who are competing to win a prize for their efforts to dramatically reduce their weight. It's clear from their speaking that their weight-losing experience is not simply about diet and exercise. Each contestant repeatedly and eloquently says, essentially, "I have become a new person. I have a new relationship with my body. I have a new relationship with food. I have a new way of seeing the world." The shift is about an internal attitudinal transformation where they bring together all the aspects of their life with a new internal observer that designs the practices for daily life – a very different approach than piecemeal tending of various aspects of the individual.

We see it happening. We see the hunger for this change in yoga centers and gyms, in the work of personal trainers, food coaches and others in the teaching role – the work of a large wellness community across America. However, most of us do not link that widespread phenomenon to shifting the expenditures of our disease-care system.

None of this is written to denigrate the important work of surgeons and medical technology. My knee works because a wonderful surgeon, an anesthesiologist, and wonderful nurses and technicians were able to put my knee back together. However, I also know that I injured that knee because I was overly tired and not being mindful.

America must right-size the demands we place on our critical care system (the system that tended my knee), our disease-care system. We will do this by moving 70-plus percent of persons who now consume the valuable time of these experts as a result of poor lifestyles out of the disease-care system, thus allowing these extraordinary people to do what they do best for the patients who really need their help.

I was amazed by the amount of detailed research presented during two days of Senate hearings on the health-care reform act in February 2009. The issue is how to bring that wealth of research into the mainstream so that what is well understood, well documented, and well known becomes part of our public policy. I believe this will happen only when it is understood that our culture can have a minimum of a $4 to $1 return on investment by shifting from the current focus on disease to a focus on wellness. And that needs to be done where appropriate. The support system for our people and the well-being of our community depend on an investment in expanding wellness.

There is no excuse for delay. The expansion of these resources must be made an urgent national priority if we are to avoid national bankruptcy generated by the uncontrolled and seemingly uncontrollable expenditure of an unfocused disease-care system. Making well-living a national priority is not merely a good thing to consider. *I say it must be an urgent priority for national security in all senses of that word.*

NOTES

1. For data and further information, see sources referenced in Essay 4, Notes 19 and 20.

2. For the full statement by Delos M. Cosgrove, MD, and further information about the Cleveland Clinic Employee Wellness Program, see www.prevent.org/data/files/initiatives/cosgrove13.pdf.

3. "Cleveland Clinic Health System; *Cleveland Clinic Employee Wellness Program.*" Summary document. Copyright © 2006 Partnership for Prevention™.

4. Information about InspireHealth and its integrative cancer care programs is available at www.inspirehealth.ca.

5. "Secrets of Happiness – Blue Zones" aired on ABC's 20/20 on January 11, 2008. The documentary is based on Dan Buettner's book, *The Blue Zones: Lessons for Living Longer From the People Who've Lived the Longest* (National Geographic, 2008}.

6. Books, articles, and videos about the Blue Zones are available at www.bluezones.com, including a DVD about Dan Buettner's travels to Ikaria and the longevity secrets of its inhabitants: "Ikaria, Greece Blue Zone." You can see the monk in a brief film on YouTube, "The Blue Zones Ikaria Quest Day 5."

7. Among numerous resources focusing on wellness:
   – Andrew Weil. *Eight Weeks to Optimum Health: A Proven Program for Taking Full Advantage of Your Body's Natural Healing Power* (Knopf, updated edition, 2006). For more resources, visit www.drweil.com.
   – James Gordon. *Manifesto for A New Medicine: Your Guide to Healing Partnerships and the Wise Use of Alternative Therapies* (Da Capo Press, 1997). For more resources, visit www.cmbm.org.
   – Dean Ornish. *Dr. Dean Ornish's Program for Reversing Heart Disease:*

The Only System Scientifically Proven to Reverse Heart Disease Without Drugs or Surgery (Ivy Books, 1995). For more resources, visit www.or-nishspectrum.com.

– Mehmet Oz. *YOU: The Owner's Manual: An Insider's Guide to the Body that Will Make You Healthier and Younger* (William Morrow, up-dated expanded edition, 2008). For more resources, visit www.doctoroz. com.

– John W. Travis. *The Wellness Workbook: How to Achieve Enduring Health and Vitality* (Celestial Arts, 3rd edition, 2004). For more resources, visit www.thewellspring.com.

– Deepak Chopra. *Reinventing the Body, Resurrecting the Soul: How to Create a New You* (Three Rivers Press, reprint edition, 2010). For more resources, visit deepakchopra.com.

8. Martin E.P. Seligman, *Flourish: A Visionary New Understanding of Happiness and Well-Being* (New York: Free Press, Division of Simon & Schuster, 2011). For resources about Dr. Seligman's work, see www.ppc. sas.upenn.edu and www.pursuit-of-happiness.org/history-of-happiness/martin-seligman.

9. Jonathan Haidt. *The Happiness Hypothesis: Finding Modern Truth in Ancient Wisdom* (Basic Books, 2006). For resources about the work of Jonathan Haidt, see www.HappinessHypothesis.com.

10. "Integrative Medicine and the Health of the Public: A Summary of the February 2009 Summit" is available at www.iom.edu.

11. Nortin Hadler, *Worried Sick: A Prescription for Health in an Overtreated America* (University of North Carolina Press, 2008), and *The Last Well Person: How to Stay Well Despite the Health-Care System* (McGill-Queen's University Press, 2007).

12. For resources about the work of Abraham Verghese, MD, see www.abra-hamverghese.com.

13. Atul Gawande, "The Hot Spotters." *The New Yorker* (January 24, 2011). For resources about the work of Atul Gawande, MD, see gawande.com.

Economics 102 – Taking Control of Your Wellness *and* Your Health-care Dollars

"We put wellness programs in two communities. It went so well, we almost closed two community hospitals for lack of admissions. We cut back on wellness."
– *Personal comment from the medical director of a major national health insurance company (after demonstrating his tai chi skills)*

"We already have medical rationing. Patients do not know the cost of care, and thus do not know how much would be available to their family if they knew how to spend their health-care dollars wisely."
– *President of a community hospital, speaking to a group of Rotarians (paraphrased)*

LEON, AN ELDERLY gentleman, came to my inner-city clinic. He suffered from diabetes, neuropathy, high blood pressure, arthritis, and many minor strokes. He was in and out of the emergency room so frequently that I joked the ambulance was on automatic to go to his house and back to the hospital.

Leon had been a successful chef in Baltimore for many years, but when the effects of diabetes set in, he could no longer work. When I began to explore his diet, I realized something was deeply amiss. It turned out he had lost his access to food stamps because his daughter was taking the stamps and selling them to buy drugs. The one who was punished for her actions was Leon, who could no longer buy healthy food and thus was eating a disastrous diet for a diabetic.

I was able to help in getting decent food into the house, and the acupuncture and coaching were helping him; but something still wasn't quite right.

Leon often talked about church, although he never attended a service. It took me several weeks to catch on, but then I had a realization. I said, "Leon, you don't go to church because you don't have a proper suit." I could tell by the look on his face that this was the reason – simply the lack of a suit.

We arranged for him to go to the Goodwill. For about fifty dollars Leon found a suit, tie, and shirt that he felt good about wearing to church. He quickly reconnected with his church community – his life support community. To my knowledge, Leon never again went to the emergency room. No longer is he dependent on the ER, the ambulance, or food stamps. His dignity has been restored. And he is no longer costing the health-care system a fortune.

Low-tech before High-tech

I was astounded in the early 1980s to encounter a report by the American Council of Life Insurance predicting the three dimensions of what the health-care system in America would look like in the year 2030:[1]

1. There would be emergency rooms to deal with accidents, trauma, extreme shock, severe illnesses, and catastrophes.

2. There would be an equivalent to what we now call ATM machines, into which you could put your finger for immediate diagnosis of blood markers. It would then immediately deliver the pills you needed to address any disease.

3. And third, most care would be returned to the family and community. As was the case with my childhood in New York City, people in the neighborhood would know ways of dealing with most diseases; and ordinary, everyday care would be largely deprofessionalized, saving the emergency-care system for true emergencies.

This vision made sense to me then and still does today – that the primary and most common level of intervention be the least invasive level of intervention, and that the individual would be aware of the wisdom of his/her body and know the commonsense ways of keeping well: herbs, diet, sleep, fluid intake, exercise, and other daily healthy patterns. This would be the normal response before looking for more technological interventions.

Self-care with Real-time Benefits before Disease Prevention

For decades, public health experts have been passionate about putting the ideal of self-care back at center stage. This approach should appeal to all policymakers, whether they are on the left or right of the political spectrum, not only because it works (as it has for millennia), but because it will free up trillions of dollars from disease-care spending, allowing the system to liberate itself from the overloads and distractions that unnecessarily clog its functioning.

This change can't happen on its own. A public dialogue must be generated, societal support must be won, and strong policy initiatives must be developed. It is a very new idea for the modern person to take responsibility for his or her own wellness and well-being when the modern person is barraged by constant television ads trumpeting the newest fashionable diseases and the most invasive medical interventions to combat them, from heart surgeries to multicolored pills. (A recent TV ad makes a local hospital complex seem like such a wonderland, I have to remind myself not to sign up to go there for my next vacation.)

We do not need more conversations about better disease prevention. We've been trying that for many years, and its effectiveness is largely offset by increased fear and increased medical spending. And most people do not respond well to feeling guilty. Our national policy focus should be about being well *and knowing how we know that we are well* by developing mindful awareness about our bodies, just as we must be aware of our bank account balance and the heat in the house and the servicing of the car and whether the meat in the fridge is still safe to eat.

The essential policy shift is a commitment to placing the lowest-tech, the lowest-cost interventions before high-tech, high-cost interventions – an approach where (in non-emergency situations, of course) the wisdom of the individual is primary and must be exhausted before expensive high-tech intervention is used.

We made progress in this area recently when the FDA urged parents of young children to limit the use of antibiotics and over-the-counter medications to when they are absolutely necessary. The parents were informed most over-the-counter drugs are not useful for the common cold and infections in small children. Unfortunately, however, the parents were not taught the natural wisdom used for centuries by mothers in such cases – wisdom used before we began medicalizing the common cold and telling parents to ignore the family wisdom and consult a modern expert. We cannot easily reverse the momentum of 50 years of "always consult the expert." It will take time and a lot of wise public education messages to shift this trend.

There is a common understanding that if you let a cold run its course, it will take a week to clear; and if you have a medical intervention, it will take a week and however many dollars. A policy that creates an awareness of this distinction in the public and educates about natural ways to ease discomfort and improve the immune system, as well as provide guidelines about when to escalate intervention – such a policy can only increase satisfaction.

Satisfaction from Understanding

In the early 1990s, I helped organize (with funding from five large Maryland corporations) anthropologic research examining the stories of more than 600 patients in six different acupuncture clinics located across America. We were not seeking to prove anything; we simply wanted to quantify how a large number of clients described what they were getting for their mostly out-of-pocket payments.

We recorded their concerns and complaints – what I call their ticket in the door to a health professional. We recorded the sense of benefit or lack of benefit they received. We invited them to write essays describing their experience. It should be noted these clinics practiced very different styles of acupuncture and were run by providers with different personalities. Probably because of self-selection, most of the respondents reported a 90 percent rate of either full or significant improvement in their symptoms.

The most interesting outcome to me, however, despite these impressive symptomatic reports, was that *in only two of the six clinics did the patients report satisfaction with their experience.* In these two clinics the patients reported satisfaction because *they had been educated to understand how they generated their symptoms.*

This outcome is echoed in an article published in *Alternative Therapies* in 2006 by Drs. Mark Stibich and Lawrence Wissow from the University of San Diego and Johns Hopkins School of Public Health, respectively. The authors report that the most significant outcome among patients was a sense of understanding – what the authors call the "meaning response" – through which people began to have power over their symptoms by observing and understanding them.[2]

Creating knowledge and empowerment in patients not only saves everyone money from not increasing the level of intervention, it also has a side-effect of happy patients. It brings a real-time benefit of well-being.

The True Physician Treats the Person

In the ancient Chinese medical texts, there is a clear distinction between the doctor who can get rid of a symptom without curing the person, the mid-level doctor who can somewhat diagnose the disease and provide great assistance, and the true physician who enables the person to heal themselves. This echoes William Osler, one of the founding professors of Johns Hopkins Hospital: *The great physician treats the person who has the disease, not the disease that has the person.*

As we have this conversation about our health-care dollars, we must realize health professionals are divided into similar groups: technicians who narrowly focus on treating symptoms and disease, and healers who look at the whole person and teach the art of wellness.

Both groups will always be essential. Now, however, we must shift the focus to expanding the role of the healer and empowering the individual to be his/her own healer in the broader sense.

In my own field, there are acupuncturists who can be quite

magical at removing symptoms. I once had a student who had practiced acupuncture in Shanghai for many years and who could make almost any symptom disappear by simple treatments. Yet her patients had to keep returning so she could keep "disappearing" the original symptoms, as well as any new symptoms that developed as a result of suppressing the "warning light" of the original "ticket," the original alerting symptom. That is a very expensive use of acupuncture; and of course, this is a pattern that appears throughout the medical profession. Not only do costs go up, but the primary responsibility for managing the care is turned over to the specialist rather than held by the informed patient. Increased costs in health care almost always follow this abdication of responsibility.

Conversely, there are other health professionals whose success ultimately comes from being wellness educators, no matter what title appears on their door. They understand that their patients have the intrinsic wisdom to live well and fully; and while this intrinsic wisdom is often ignored, it can be rediscovered and applied when the patient is asked the right questions and given the right coaching. In this way, the overall person is helped and the "warning light" symptoms go out on their own, without being masked by unnecessary medications and treatments.

This is a different kind of health professional, one who does not create a dependency on his/her own services and interventions, instead awakening the curiosity of patients about what they can do to help themselves. In the presence of a chronic illness, these teacher-healers provoke understanding in their patients about how they can shift their habits to manage their condition and wisely make use of high-tech professional expertise. When serious illness and death approach, they sensitively guide their patients into designing a process that maximizes the quality of their remaining life. (This is very different from the expert who will fight to prolong life, no matter what the consequences, costs, or wishes of the patient.)

As a matter of national policy, we need to understand this

distinction between "fixing the symptom" and guiding patients to support their own well-being – and we need to find ways to talk about it. In my teaching I refer to it as a "deal" between the patient and the practitioner: Is the agreement for a quick fix that will have to be repeated ad infinitum, or is it for long-term understanding of ways of living well that will minimize problems to begin with? It's like repeatedly engaging a mechanic who is happy to keep taking your money to fix the brakes on your car, versus one who will show you a way of driving that avoids the damage in the first place.

Generating this intrinsic understanding is critical because true wellness is not expert-driven; it is driven and understood by the individual; it is an inner state versus a set of techniques. Knowing and eating foods that have me feel well is very different from my following the prescribed norms of someone else's image of wellness. Perhaps it's necessary that a professional guide me in learning to notice and appreciate how my body responds. And once I have this skill, it is mine for life.

A Generational Change

This shift may take generations. And we must start now. We are dealing with an updated version of the old adage, "Give a man a fish and you feed him for a day; teach a man to fish and you feed him for a lifetime." It will be easier to develop these habits with the next generations than with people who are steeped in our current model.

Right now, however, there is much that can be given to enhance the quality of life for the elderly. It is well-documented that elderly people who do tai chi every day have fewer falls and therefore, on the whole, generate far less costs for hip or leg surgery. So by doing tai chi every day, they deprive acupuncturists of income, deprive surgeons of income, deprive the insurance, hospital, and pharmaceutical systems of income. By paying a few dollars to a tai chi teacher, they help to balance our federal budget by reducing the number of surgeries paid for by Medicare. More importantly for these people, they report a heightened sensory awareness of the world around them. They learn to breathe more deeply and be more accepting of life, thus reducing their levels of stress and stress-induced illness and improving their overall experience of being alive.

I wonder what will emerge when, instead of beginning to teach this sort of practice to senior citizens, it is taught to first graders. Imagine the effects of mindful breathing and simple yoga movements for teachers and young students and their parents. It has been shown academic scores improve in classes that start with brief moments of stretching and deep breathing. Imagine the impact on health-care costs for this extended group of people over a lifetime. Imagine the impact that a generation with increased awareness and sense of aliveness will have on the health-care costs of the next generations.

My own adult children – who are alive and well! – were raised with similar teachings and have rarely visited a physician outside of the required school medical exams. They are living examples of well-living as its own reward, both in its impact on their quality of life and on their wallets. And all of us have lower health-care costs and are less burdensome to society as a whole.

The End of the Conundrum of the Iron Triangle of Cost, Quality, Access

This approach, at its heart, focuses on expanding wellness on a daily basis, and enjoying its real-time rewards instead of waiting around to fight disease when it develops. It is so simple that it can be understood intrinsically by the first grader and senior citizen alike. However, this sort of awareness is quite foreign to those of us who were not raised with it, or who have not been lucky enough to encounter a teacher-healer in the guise of a physician. Interestingly, it may be familiar to those who tune in on Oprah Winfrey's show when she has guests like Mehmet Oz, MD, sharing his simple ways to promote life-long wellness. Oprah herself is a master example of someone generating wealth and customer satisfaction via her philosophy of individual empowerment and self-inquiry.

Thirty years ago, a wise healer, Ted Kaptchuk, now an associate professor at Harvard, described this approach to me in terms of a circle:

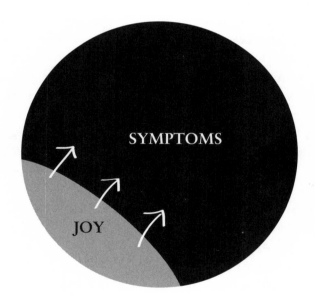

In the above circle the "symptoms" are just that: the manifestations of pathology. The "joy" is whatever a person enjoys doing: dancing, watching baseball, playing music. The healer helps individuals expand the areas of life they enjoy, and in that process recover power over the pathology by enhancing the quality of their life. Imagine the "joy" quarter of the circle expanding, crowding out their perception of misery.

The economics of this approach are vastly different from those that confound us today. The iron triangle of the cost, quality, access conundrum is no longer applicable. From this perspective, health insurance recovers its appropriate role in supporting us through the unexpected and catastrophic events of life: accidents, serious pathologies and disease. Without that insurance-conversation involved with every minor ailment, we do not have to pathologize, label, and code all of the pains and sufferings of life. We can take the funding we use in the medicalization of our existence and redirect those funds to living fully. This will mean a loss for the pharmaceutical company and an increase in cash income for the theater owner – or the racetrack, or the cruise line, or the local gym, or massage therapist, or yoga teacher. This is what a shift in funds from a focus on pathology to a focus on wellness would mean as part of our national economy.

What about rationing access to medical services?

We already have extensive medical rationing in the most irrational of ways. The shift I am proposing ends the worry of medical rationing. As the overall health-care system is used more appropriately, the resources for the truly important and essential services will be freed up and more available to all. The doctors, nurses, technicians, and receptionists also will be more satisfied and able to listen, to restore humanity and healing to what has commonly become a highly technical, dehumanized experience. Because many fewer persons will require access to the high-tech system, the physician will be able to spend more than seven minutes with each individual.

What about "my doctor"? What will happen to her?

Access to medical care (disease care) will look a lot like it does today. Insurance will cover the cost as usual. The medical staff will have more time to focus carefully on the needs of each person. And all disease care will occur in the cultural context of wellness support. For example, the care of a cancer patient naturally will include wellness education and coaching as well as access to the appropriate complementary modalities such as acupuncture or herbs or meditation. We have operating examples of this approach to health care; I think especially of the InspireHealth Clinics in Vancouver, Canada, described in Essay 9.

How do I pay for wellness?

As this shift occurs, dollars you now spend directly for health insurance and for out-of-pocket co-pays (and even more significantly, dollars your employer diverts from your salary into the corporate payments for health insurance) will begin to stay in your pocket, or begin to appear in increased wages. I wrote an article many years ago describing a family on a vacation in Hawaii, a vacation totally paid for by rebates from the non-use of their health-care dollars, hence effectively diverting funds from the disease-care industry to the Hawaii tourist and airline industries – industries that generate happiness and pleasure and thus wellness.

Who pays for wellness for the poor?

Society already pays for medicalized disease care for the poor. And society does this in the least efficient and most expensive way. Programs will be designed to divert dollars from disease care to wellness care; I believe venture capitalists will be happy to enable this transition in return for an appropriate share of the annual savings.

How will I pay for acupuncture and herbs, massage, yoga, and the many other professionalized forms of care?

Society increasingly will understand the role of these techniques in maximizing the effectiveness and reducing the overall cost of high-tech care in the treatment of disease: These techniques support the inner wellness of the person receiving highly invasive and yet essential interventions. Again, a classic demonstration is the work of InspireHealth in Canada in bringing all these skills together to produce greater patient satisfaction. When there is disease, the insurers will pay to maximize the availability of natural care, if for no other reason than to reduce the amount and cost of high-tech interventions required for patient satisfaction.

Most natural medicine will be paid for out-of-pocket as part of "good living." Theater tickets are good for you. Golf is good for you. Dance is good for you. All are paid for out-of-pocket. Massage and acupuncture are good for you; and they help you grow in your awareness of what it means to keep yourself well. So all this is a normal expense of life. The funds will be available to you because of greatly reduced disease-care costs; they are, effectively, rebates from current health insurance levels – funds being restored to you. They never should have been taken from you in the first place.

What is the role of the "health savings accounts"?

Health savings accounts and other tax structures can be designed to enhance the speed of transition to a wellness culture; and these tax incentives will and must be offset by the reduced expenditure of tax dollars on disease care.

How will our national corporations pay for wellness programming?

Businesses already are realizing the benefits of wellness programs. Corporations such as Dow Chemical and many others have discovered that investing in employee wellness delivers a direct return to the corporate bottom line of between $3 and $6 for every dollar spent on wellness. In addition, they reap the benefits of a happier, more energized workforce with significantly lower absenteeism and employee turnover.

I believe the delivery of most of these programs still occurs at a rather primitive level. Most programs are focused mainly on prevention of known disease patterns and not yet on empowerment of individuals and quality of life.

What happens to the current insurance system and diagnostic codes?

The current system will continue at a much more appropriate size. These businesses will "right-size" themselves in the same way the medical and pharmaceutical industries will be appropriately right-sized. The necessary downward trajectory of the businesses will be mitigated somewhat by the rapid growth of aging populations and a corresponding increase in the need for access to acute care.

The smart entrepreneurial components of these industries will quickly redesign themselves as providers of wellness service . . . and many of them already have begun to do so.

WIN WIN WIN! More Access and Better Quality at a Lower Cost

By asking a different set of questions, we achieve the remarkable outcome of breaking the seemingly impossible conundrum of cost, quality, and access. We expand access and quality by shifting the focus of the dollars invested in health care. Thus a WIN WIN WIN for all – empowerment for individuals, families, corporations, and the taxpayer, and a national sense of pride and accomplishment.

NOTES

1. Trend Analysis Program Report, #19, published by the American Council of Life Insurance, 1850 K Street, NW, Washington, DC, 20006.

2. Mark Stibich and Lawrence Wissow, "Meaning shift: findings from wellness acupuncture." *Alternative Therapies in Health and Medicine* (March/April 2006, Volume 12, No. 2).

A GRAND CHALLENGE

$100 Million Prize

Imagine if Apple or Google or IBM or the US Government were to offer a $100 million cash prize to any group that successfully demonstrated a reduction of more than 20 percent in absolute healthcare costs for a self-insured US corporation with more than 10,000 employees, while at the same time achieving lower employee hospitalizations, lower pharmaceutical usage, lower absenteeism, lower employee turnover, and higher employee satisfaction.

For large a corporation such as Apple or Google or IBM, offering such a prize would be self-funding within a few years. For example, I've estimated Apple Inc.'s employee health-care expenditures at more than $320 million per year: $8,000 for each of the more than 40,000 US based employees and an expense line that is presumably growing at rate of 4+ percent, or more than $12 million per year.

A successful challenge would enable a company such as Apple to offer such a proven wellness program to its employees and thus save an estimated $50 million per year from health care focused expenditures.

Not only will the company awarding the prize receive a quick return on its investment, but it also will have also created a solution with the potential to save the entire US economy!

Entrepreneurial Initiatives *for* Our Nation

"Change only takes place through action.
Not through prayer or meditation, but through action."
– The Dalai Lama

"Health care today is not meant to be a business. It is meant to be
a transformational endeavor grounded in the day-to-day needs
of people. We must all think of ourselves as patient advocates.
We must advocate for prevention and wellness. We must fight for
integrative health care. We need to change the health-care system
from a 'sick-care' system to a true 'health-care' system."
– Senator Barbara Mikulski, Member, US Senate Committee on
Health, Education, Labor, and Pensions; Chair, Subcommittee on
Children and Families

MY MOTHER-IN-LAW, June Eliott, provides an
illustrative case study about modern health care. June is now 86
years old and doing very well. When her husband died 13 years

ago, my wife, Susan, arranged for her to live near us. When June arrived, Susan found her a physician who practiced internal medicine. The doctor provided wonderful service for my mother-in-law, who had few problems and took very few medications under her care. About four years ago, her doctor announced she was going to limit the size of her practice. The physician's practice was so successful that it became overloaded, and she decided to provide care to a limited number of individuals who would have to sign up for a "boutique package" at a charge of $150 each month, a charge that provided for extraordinary care and accessibility. When her doctor talked to June about joining this plan, June said, "I don't see you very much, and I don't need much care, so I don't see much value in paying that extra money. I really care about you and appreciate your service, but I think I will see someone else." That was fine with everyone, and the doctor referred June to the physician who was taking her place in the general practice.

After about a year and a half with her new physician, Susan noticed June was being sent for tests almost every month and was visiting the hospital for MRIs – one thing after another. She was becoming a regular visitor to doctors' offices and the hospital; she was on more and more medications; and she was feeling less well and less happy. As Susan became of aware of what was happening, she suggested June needed a geriatrician, a doctor who would understand the issues of aging and would also understand the dangers of over-medication and over-testing. Throughout this phase, June often said to us, "With all this testing, even if they find something, I don't want any great invasive treatments. I've lived a good life, and I don't want massive interventions of any sort."

As most folks do, June has a respect for doing what her doctor tells her and would say "yes" to whatever was asked of her. On the other hand, she was blessed to have a daughter like Susan, who understood the many options in health care and was not caught in the monopoly mode of "this is the only alternative." Susan began to inquire about other physicians and found Dr. Andy Lazris in Columbia, Maryland. The first thing this wise doctor did was to spend a long time talking to June, asking her a lot of questions, and eventually taking her off many of her medications. He asked her, "Do you want a lot of testing, or shall we just keep you comfortable for the rest of your years?" Suddenly June was feeling brighter and stronger, on fewer medications, and made the decision to move into a retirement village where Dr. Lazris happened to be the physician. She is now more active than she's been for many years.

The significance of June's story for our discussion about the economics of health care is that because she doesn't need those many services, she no longer costs Medicare or her private insurance backup very much money. Extrapolate the amount saved in June's example by 80 to 90 percent of the people in Medicare. Train health-care providers to listen and more open-mindedly tend life's difficult issues, as did Dr. Lazris, and we will move billions of dollars from the negative disease-care column into the wellness column.

Preparing our nation for a wellness-based future requires two main activities: encouraging entrepreneurs to seek profits from investing in wellness programs, and ending regulations and habits that unwittingly support the current monopoly.

Background

In 1974, Maryland was the only state in our country with a firm law that allowed the practice of acupuncture, although there was one major specification: "provided there is medical supervision." Many other states had opinions from their medical boards that were less hospitable to my discipline and mostly very restrictive. And so I moved to Maryland.

Upon my arrival, the medical doctors who agreed to provide supervision were immediately threatened by the Maryland Board of Medical Examiners with the loss of their licenses because "regulations defining supervision have not yet been issued." This began a long, complicated, and very expensive adventure (and introduction for me to the idea of $200-per-hour legal fees!), which to most Americans now seems absurd. And yet it was the natural outcome of the 1908 Flexner Report that led to non-allopathic forms of health care becoming illegal.

Although we acupuncturists eventually prevailed, almost four decades later Maryland still doesn't have laws celebrating and protecting the rights of those who provide herbal remedies or homeopathic preparations, or even of those who are asked to provide an at-home reflexology treatment to a neighbor. The NIH Center for Complementary and Alternative Medicine has identified more than 200 distinct forms of healing considered outside the mainstream of American medicine that might ease or prevent suffering in Maryland's citizens. While acupuncture is now legal in my state (and to be sure, the acupuncture profession is now generating its own turf battles against other professions), the monopolistic cultural and legal stance remains in place.

Changing that restrictive stance into a cultural celebration of diversity must now become a primary interest of government. Government must restore the primary responsibility for health and wellness to the individual and to the family. Today, our nation has an urgent vested interest in making individuals their own primary care provider and ending destructive turf wars, an approach that will allow well-informed persons to choose among many effective options in their own community.

Many components of a community-level wellness system are already in place in the United States. This must be acknowledged and celebrated in order to break the conundrum of the iron triangle: cost-access-quality (Essays 3 and 5). The United States has an enormous number of wellness providers in the form of holistically-oriented massage therapists, acupuncturists, nutritionists, naturopaths, herbalists, chiropractors, physicians, and nurses. Many of these providers are licensed, and an even larger number are self-educated and use their healing skills for friends and neighbors and family, much as my parents and grandparents knew the basics of living well and tending to those with illness.

Wonderful practitioners are often constrained from truly holistic service by the turf battles that rage within and around their professions. For example, I've been told I cannot recommend to patients that they drink more water because that is the province of nutritionists. In many states some of these professions work to protect their turf from the growing army of lay herbalists and homeopaths who easily could be arrested for "practicing medicine without a license."

When they do thrive, wellness practitioners such as myself also are constrained by the concepts of insurance that require them to categorize their patients in terms of coded diseases. Many practitioners do not feel valuable unless they are recognized for insurance reimbursement. I remember an NIH meeting where a group of yoga teachers wanted to be recognized as health professionals for insurance purposes. Yoga is a way of life in much of the world, not a medical technique, yet our culture is on the edge of twisting yoga into a medicalized tool instead of a pleasurable habit.

An even bigger natural resource for a new wellness world are the thousands of individuals who teach wellness but are called clerks in the herb aisle of Whole Foods, or are fitness trainers at the gym. There is also the rapidly growing profession of wellness coaches.

Readiness for the wellness-based healing culture is also exemplified by the national eagerness for and receptiveness to teachings about natural medicine and home-healing that are staples of the Dr. Oz show and Oprah's OWN channel.

Policies that focus on wellness promotion also promote

increased employment. Wellness is a high-touch, low-tech industry. It is labor intensive rather than machine intensive. It is not an "assembly-line" approach to healing; rather it is actively personal.

Thus a wellness focus brings many benefits to our economy and our nation as a whole.

I suggest a series of national initiatives to incentivize a shift in assumptions about health and health care at little or no cost to governments, insurers, or corporations – initiatives at every level enabling a shift from a set of cultural assumptions that have brought us to the brink of disaster, both economically and in terms of the wellness of our community, and that offer little hope for the wellness of future generations.

The health-care deck is stacked by advertising that generates widespread fear, by advertising that disempowers the wisdom of the body and promotes a dependency on expert advice and pharmaceuticals, advertising that discourages an individual from looking at the totality of his or her life situation and narrowly focuses on specialized parts, not taking the whole person into account.

These new wellness initiatives have a sense of urgency and are essential to restoring dignity and hope.

These recommendations do not challenge the need for the existing emergency room and critical care system, an essential system and true benefit of the last 50 years of technology and medicine. The critical care system must be left in place. The doctors, nurses, and technicians who are part of that system will be used appropriately, focusing their skills on the emergency and pathological situations for which they were highly trained, and – this the key point – they will not be distracted by the 80 percent of patients who are better served in a much more organic, simple, low-tech way. These proposals in no way challenge the use of surgery and pharmaceuticals when appropriate and essential. Likewise, they in no way promote a fight with the existing health-care system, which provides core services highly beneficial and important to our society.

The initiatives I propose here are conceived to provide breathing room for the existing system, allowing it to smoothly right-size itself and come into a realistic proportion with what best serves its own functioning, the national budget, and the well-being of all Americans, bringing full access, reasonable cost, and high quality. These initiatives will enable our highly capable disease-care system to focus completely on what it does best.

Furthermore, these proposals in no way privilege any form of alternative/integrated medicine over mainstream medicine. Each of the gifts brought by the many different forms of medicine are unique, and none should be favored over the other. As indicated in the previous chapters, these policies rely on an assumption that individuals have (or can have, with learning) the ability to recover their natural, god-given capacity to know how to care for themselves and for those in their families, except in the most extraordinary circumstances; and we must return that right to them.

As a young acupuncturist in England, I was struck that I could practice without a license or even a certificate. Anyone could come to me for treatment even if I didn't have a credential. However, if I wanted to work on a horse, I had to have a license and special approval because it was understood a horse couldn't review my credentials. Anyone could open a practice on Harley Street to do brain surgery because it was assumed thoughtful patients would question the credentials of anyone to whom they were about to turn over their body; and in the case of persons incompetent to make such queries, it was assumed guardians or family members would provide the necessary protection.

This story from England points to the philosophical shift underlying the initiatives presented here. Each of these recommendations reflects a shift from a dependency on experts to the empowerment of the unique individual and his or her family and community.

In a previous age, it may have been arguable this was an unwise policy because the patient could not access the necessary information and guidance. However, we now live in the twenty-first century; and as the Internet has made possible the velvet revolutions in Northern Africa, the same connectivity has furthered the empowerment of the individual to access resources about how to stay well and appropriately apply the expertise of medical and many other health professionals, as well as the advice of friends and colleagues whom they respect.

With all this in mind, I recommend that the United States (and the State of Maryland as a model for the nation) as soon as possible initiate wellness policies and pass legislation where necessary, encouraging and enabling each of the following:

Encourage Entrepreneurial Investment

1. *States can enhance the wellness of employees and their families, thus saving millions of dollars in tax money and providing a model for the nation.* Every level of government has the opportunity for enormous savings by lowering the costs of providing health care – and this can be done while enhancing the wellness of the work force. Lower costs, higher satisfaction, lower employee turnover.

Those potential benefits, as illustrated by the results at Dow Chemical and the Cleveland Clinic, can generate substantial savings for taxpayers, profits to the entrepreneurs, and happier and healthier agency employees serving the public good. The benefits occur not only in dollars *not* spent, but in reduced absenteeism and attrition, and in enhanced employee happiness. I believe happiness equals wellness and good health.

A triple bottom-line: Win-Win-Win! *And* a long-term cultural benefit for our nation.

This goal is best accomplished by inviting entrepreneurs to propose the delivery of wellness services, entirely at the entrepreneurs' expense, for willing state agencies such as the State Department of

Health, or the teachers and staff in a city or county school system, or the National Guard. Data show a minimum return on such investment of $3 for every $1 invested. These savings could be split 50/50 between the agency and investors.

2. *States can model enhancing wellness for their employees, not only as a benefit to productivity, but also as a way of saving taxpayer dollars. They also can incentivize private corporations to invest in similar initiatives.* American corporations are at an international competitive disadvantage due to being responsible for health-care costs that in every other country are not a corporate expense burden. States that encourage a shift in this cost structure will develop a culture that attracts the most capable workforce for their economic growth. This is demonstrated by the efforts of companies such as Dow Chemical, by work in positive psychology developed by Martin Seligman (see *Flourish*), and by the adoption of such principles by the US Army.

3. *Adding wellness programs to the health-care benefits of our school teachers* will be well-received emotionally ("the system is paying attention to me and helping me relieve my work-induced stress"), save health-care dollars, reduce absenteeism, and enhance employee retention. Perhaps more importantly for society, as teachers use these principles for their own well-being, they will begin to model these behaviors for parents and children, thus instigating a wide societal benefit without extra cost . . . and indeed, as noted above, with a return of at least $3 for every $1 invested in the health-care costs of teachers. This is an example of how the principle of shifting expenditures toward wellness, when rolled out strategically to those who have significant societal influence, can make a wide impact on society.

4. *States must apply these same principles to the management of*

Medicare and Medicaid services and incentivize the providers to profit from the cost savings of wellness projects . . . the profits to be shared with the government. This is the same idea as in the previous recommendations. The Penn North project in Baltimore and many similar projects are very effective at keeping people out of emergency rooms. However, the enormous cost savings generated by those projects do not cycle back into the promotion of more such programs. In demonstrations mentioned earlier involving school teachers, state agencies, and private corporations, we can track the cost savings and see the project's direct value. Not so with Medicare and Medicaid. Because they are funded on a diagnostic disease model, their payments are made per procedure and per intervention. With a lack of alignment of goals and outcome measurements, the cycle of financial benefit is not demonstrated, and the cash cannot recycle to where it has the highest impact on the quality of life for individuals and reduces costs to the overall system. This must change. Alignment of outcomes is essential – an alignment where both medical groups and community groups benefit by tending the well-being of the whole person and the whole community.

5. Maryland should immediately model for the nation a StateStat for health, as it has done already for crime, addictions, the environmental care of the Chesapeake Bay, etc. StateStat would identify, in real time, individuals who are costing our health-care system amounts far beyond the norm, and direct specially trained persons toward these individuals. In this way, the State might identify the top two percent of individuals on whom we expend the most, and target those individuals for consultation with wellness coaches. Such an approach is highlighted by Atul Gawande, MD. (See "Hot Spotters" in the *New Yorker,* January 24, 2011). It is clear from cases noted in the article and in the work of Peter Beilenson, MD, in Howard County, Maryland, the return on investment for such a targeted state system would more than pay for itself.

Shift Our Laws and Leadership Speaking Patterns

6. *Enact health freedom legislation* enabling every individual to be his or her own primary-care provider and act as a wellness provider to fellow community members, either for free or for pay. Such legislation would end turf protection for many professionals, who would provide their services on an equal basis with everyone else. Individuals would choose providers based on the strength of the credentials, recommendations, and other available information about anyone offering services.

Such legislation has already passed in Minnesota, California, Rhode Island, and other states. Essentially, the legislation specifies that anyone may offer himself/herself to provide healing and wellness services to any other individual, for free or for pay, with certain provisos including signed consent, referral points of information, and a guarantee there has been no fraudulent presentation of skills or abilities. This legislation includes wise limitations regarding the prescribing of drugs, the performance of surgery, and of highly technical procedures that may have serious side effects – again, an emphasis on the lower-cost, low-tech interventions before more high-tech procedures. This legislation is a first step toward ending the turf battles. It would require wise judgment to identify the limited areas in which legislative restriction is required. (*Note that acupuncture is an example of a low-tech service which, due to a variety of political forces, became professionalized and thus a competing professional system, not part of the structure of ordinary life as it is in much of Asia.*)

Such health-freedom legislation would make available a diversity of health-care modalities and would end the modern monopoly of the allopathic and pharmaceutical traditions. It also would end the growing competition among naturopaths, herbalists, acupuncturists, and others for "turf control." Essentially, this legislation will release a great entrepreneurial force in our nation.[1]

7. *Protect the use of low-tech forms of care before high-tech.* This demands an understanding that much of our current cost structure is related to unnecessary testing due to fear of legal reprisal. As we have warnings on drugs about potential side effects, perhaps patients must be warned that using high-tech medicine before low-tech also has dangers. A recent example of such risk is routine PSA testing, which after being strongly recommended for all men for years has been determined to be dangerous.[2]

Similarly, using the case study of my mother-in-law, June, at the beginning of this essay, we find the physician who increasingly referred June for so much high-tech testing had never opened a conversation with her about what she would do if a test came back positive for serious disease. Would she accept high-tech interventions to postpone death? We can assume the physician acted from her best knowledge, but was focused on utilizing the available technology, not on what would benefit the patient in front of her.

When June's new physician had a conversation with her about her desires and her attitude about preventing death and the process of dying, the pattern of intervention totally changed. This conversation saved Medicare and her secondary corporate insurance provider thousands of dollars.

Our present liability system rewards providers for immediate intervention with high-tech testing. This is not sustainable. I know a wonderful physician who stopped practicing after he was successfully sued for prescribing a less-invasive medication before a more invasive medication. The result was a delay of approximately ten days in the full recovery of the patient from a mild symptom. This is at the heart of the issue of expensive testing and high-tech interventions. The conventional debate over tort reform is really a coded conversation in which we all avoid this core issue. We are not aware that we also place ourselves at greater risk with unnecessary and unwise enhanced early-stage interventions.

There must be incentives for limiting tests to procedures with direct benefit. If individuals wish additional testing, they would pay for it in full or make a significant co-pay for anything beyond the minimum recommended tests.

8. *Everyone listening . . . fostering curiosity.* One of the public's major complaints about the current health-care system is very simple: "Nobody listens." I assert this is because health-care providers are not trained to listen. Continuing medical education for any licensed provider must mandate providers be trained in wellness coaching, listening, and conversation skills. Professional leaders must emphasize the importance of this personalized connection and the importance of allowing time in the schedules of health professionals for listening, coaching, and conversation. The seven-minute office visit is inherently not cost-effective from any perspective.

9. *Conversations about dying and death.* Hospitals (and, I believe, most states) mandate patients prepare "advanced directives" – directives about how the patient wishes to be tended in the presence of serious illness and the proximity of death. These are now done mostly "pro forma": another form in the stack. And yet, it may be the most important form of all. My clinical experience and extensive academic research indicates that most professional health-care providers are not comfortable with conversations about their own mortality. A distortion of the facts about such conversations arose during the 2009 congressional health-care debate, when there was an outcry about "death panels" at a hospital where such conversations had been in place successfully for many years, providing enhanced satisfaction for patients and families and at the same time lowering system costs. Self-awareness is essential for teaching others to prepare for death, and there is no conversation more critical to shifting the practice of health and wellness in America. Well-trained specialized teams are a great gift to patients, their families, and to all.

The idea of death as an evil to be avoided at all costs is the most destructive of our basic assumptions. Professional associations must include such a recognition in their continuing-education requirements, and our national leaders must become comfortable with having such conversations in the public forum.

10. *Pharmacists as teachers.* Pharmacists should be encouraged to return to the era when the pharmacist was the local wellness coach, the teacher of simple wellness at the community level. Many pharmacists are indicating an interest; they are developing the skills to become wellness coaches, a role they already fill without specific training for that kind of informational service. We can build on this movement within the pharmaceutical profession. Wellness coaching skills bring an advantage to local pharmacists, who have been squeezed by the increasing sale of pharmaceuticals via the internet. In the future, the profit margin for the local pharmacist may have to come from the added-value service of their ability to be wellness educators – educators about the appropriate use of medications, the need for lifestyle enhancement, and the need to reduce dependency on medications.

It might become standard practice that no prescription be filled without a conversation about the importance of sleep, diet, and exercise, and that when the prescription is renewed, the pharmacist requests a report from the patient or receives a special note from the physician indicating the patient is appropriately tending such lifestyle issues. This is the place where the dangerous illusion of a "magic pill" (another of our most destructive assumptions) could encounter an enriching conversation about how changing our daily life habits might help us avoid the expense and side effects of the medication while enhancing our sense of empowerment about our quality of life.

11. *Flu vaccinations as an opportunity for wellness education.* The

annual vaccination campaign might be linked to a one-minute conversation about the importance of helping to avoid the flu by life habits that enhance our immune system through diet, exercise, sleep, and the basics of deep breathing. Imagine the long-term benefits in health and reduction in costs if every person who received a vaccination were taught the art of belly breathing and the benefits of extra sleep when they are feeling vulnerable to infection. Similar instruction should be a part of all TV commercials, vaccinations, pamphlets, public-health seminars, and related public-service campaigns.

12. *Leaders in all aspects of public life must begin to shift their background understanding of life.* Instead of speaking of life as highly stressed and oriented to financial attainment, they must begin to speak more about life as something to be enjoyed in community, pointing out that slowing the pace of life will provide real wisdom and solve many issues before they become problems, either medical problems or behavioral problems in the community. They must speak of the wisdom of taking time to enjoy life; enjoying basketball, walking, or eating well can be presented as good in themselves. We must replace stress as the cultural badge of honor with recognition that life well-lived is the most important yardstick of success.

We should enjoy living! Going for a walk should not be done simply to avoid a heart attack, but because walking is a wonderful source of pleasure in itself. With this, we must find ways to speak effectively of the individual as his/her own primary-care provider. The outside expert may be essential for infectious and communicable diseases and accidents; however, in caring for the non-communicable, lifestyle-generated diseases that dominate our modern world, individuals must recover their own power.

Conclusion

Encouraging such policies and specific demonstration projects in state agencies, corporations, school systems, and Medicare and Medicaid will engender a national flow of copycat initiatives in the private sector based on the opportunity for a significant return on investment – programs such as those being implemented in British Columbia and Vancouver with regard to cancer (described in Essay 9); the programs in England incentivizing physicians to incorporate natural care in their practice; and programs in companies already seeing a dollar return of three-to-one on their investment in the wellness of employees.

When the initiatives suggested above are operational, they will serve as models that slowly generate a ripple effect as leaders see the savings in taxpayer funds and the benefits to individuals. Such a model will transform what now is considered extraordinary behavior into the ordinary way of life. The resources already existing within our diverse systems will be used appropriately by a population beginning to take back the power to design its own wellness and health care.

Basing new actions on new assumptions provides a way to end forever the usual political discourse about the impossibility of the iron triangle of cost-quality-access – a false conundrum and a destructive conversation.

There is nothing really novel about the wellness proposals in these essays. As I come to the end of this writing, I read in the *Los Angeles Times* of the death, at age 97, of Lester Breslow, MD, referred to by many as "Mr. Public Health." In 1959, Dr. Breslow identified seven habits of healthy living: regular exercise, regular sleep, not smoking, moderate use of alcohol, eating regularly (including breakfast), and maintaining a normal weight. He documented that those who followed these seven habits increased their life expectancy by eleven years as compared to those who followed fewer than four of the habits. It is time for Americans to make these basic habits part of the national culture, thus increasing their quality of life and decreasing the overwhelming costs of health care.[3]

Our nation is worthy of large-minded national discourse. These conversations and existing demonstrations must now be elevated to center stage in our national arena. To avoid enhancing this discourse is to risk national bankruptcy. This wellness conversation, this quality-of-life conversation, is now ready for the national stage.

NOTES

1. For information about health freedom legislation, see www.national-healthfreedom.org.

2. For more about the risks of over-medicalization, see Nortin M. Hadler, *The Last Well Person: How to Stay Well Despite the Health-care System* (McGill-Queens University Press, 2004).

3. Lester Breslow. *Autobiography: A Life in Public Health: An Insider's Retrospective* (Springer Publishing Company, 2004).

I Commit Myself

The Dalai Lama reminds us, "Change only takes place through action." Action requires that somebody do the action. Thus as I complete these essays, I commit myself:

- To be available to interested leaders, linking them with the resources that enable them to be cultural change agents for self-care and cutting the costs of health care.

- To be available to mentor those who are committed to recovering their own wellness and teaching others the skills for self-care.

- And, over 2012–2013, to empower . . .

100 families – parents, grandparents, children – learning together in cohorts of six or seven families. Guided by an experienced wellness mentor, these families recover their to ability to live well – to cook together, to know how to select good food, develop excellent exercise habits, learn skills for coping with the everyday colds and fevers, pains and aches of human life without unnecessarily consulting the experts.

Together, they recover wise ways of dealing with the stages of life: childbirth, raising children, guiding young adults, tending relationships, and tending the elders in the most family-friendly ways possible. In the process, at the family dinner table they will pass along to their children this wisdom about how to live well, as has been the habit of humans for centuries.

They will learn about breathing, stretching, yoga, family massage. They will gain basic skills in using herbs and homeopathic remedies for everyday illnesses. And they will be much more informed in determining when it is essential to consult a physician or head to the emergency room, and when they do so, how to interact effectively.

They will learn language skills to communicate effectively with minimum stress, learn how to coordinate the chores of life – getting the dishes done and the children to bed. They will have skills enabling them to avoid the stresses and expectations that generate so much unnecessary pain.

All of This Will Be Developed Through:

1. Monthly afternoon and evening gatherings in which families learn, cook, and eat together, guided by an experienced healer/ wellness coach.

2. Seasonal one-day learning conferences shared by many families engaged in similar learning, with workshops led by pediatricians, gerontologists, herbalists, great cooks, etc.

3. Practical resources, such as books and videos recommended to deepen their learning, discussed in study groups.

4. The deepest learning occurs as they share their teachings with other families.

The Mentors

The healers and wellness coaches will spend a full day each month studying together and preparing to enrich their cohort of families.

The 100 Families program leader: Bob Duggan

Cost

Each family will pay a modest fee each month to be part of this learning experience.

I expect the wisdom learned by each family will spread quickly to several related families.

APPENDIX B

The American Wellness System: An Alternative Way of Thinking

By Robert Duggan, MA, MAc

Statement at Hearing of the US Senate Committee on Health, Education, Labor, and Pensions

February 23, 2009

"The significant problems that we have cannot be solved at the same level of thinking we were at when we created them."
– *Albert Einstein*

The usual conversation about the American health-care system revolves around what is called "the iron triangle of cost-quality-access." In reality, a change in any one of these aspects will affect all the others. We suggest that the "iron triangle" presents a false dilemma, and that this level of thinking cannot solve the current crisis.

We must incentivize 75 percent of people to move from the current sick-care system to a self-pay, community-focused wellness system.

Preamble: How We Got in this Situation

1. The United States has a sick-care system, a disease-prevention system, and a death-prevention system – all of this with great expense and very little public satisfaction. (I cite an NIH official, Ezekiel Emanuel, writing in JAMA, May 15, 2007.)

2. A 60-year focus on turning to experts to fix disease has effectively taken away the capacity of the individual and the family to know how to tend their own symptoms and diseases. The automatic refrain, "Ask your doctor before you do anything," has created a massive feeling of impotency throughout the public.

3. This disempowerment of the public originates with the Flexner Report in 1908. Devised essentially at Johns Hopkins, the study resulted in the closing of most other schools of healing by 1920. Thus the ascendancy of what we currently call "medicine" was actually crafted 100 years ago in a process that greatly reduced the diversity of healing options.

4. The longing for expert-based care was advanced by the discoveries of antibiotics and blood transfusions and other acknowledged miracles of modern medicine. It was assumed as with many other aspects of life, that everything could be made well by technology. In the last quarter of the 20th century, this myth began to recede; and now the plea of the American public is a simple call to the medical profession: "Please listen."

5. Several studies at Tai Sophia indicate that even when symptoms are relieved, patients often are not satisfied. Satisfaction is correlated with "I now understand how I control my symptoms." Having an expert remove a headache is a vastly

different experience than having someone teach you how to change your own headache by drinking more water, getting more sleep, breathing more deeply, or clearing an upset. (The research of Nortin Hadler, MD, Claire Cassidy, PhD, and others underscore this observation.)

6. A root of this issue is an assumption long held in the medical community that the mind and the body are separate, and that the physical body can be dealt with separately from dealing with emotions – a view that now is clearly unsustainable from a scientific perspective.

7. The situation for health care is similar to the issue of creating a sustainable planet. Humans must learn to live appropriately and well with our bodies, tending life as it is. In both cases, the issue is sustainability.

8. Almost all existing conversations about health policy – whether mainstream or complementary or integrative – focus inherently on treating disease, preventing disease, and preventing death. All of the economic incentives go to those who claim to tend these aspects of health care; and insurance reimbursement is linked to the identification of the disease being treated, the disease being prevented, or the particular cause of death.

Resources: Building on a Movement Already Well in Place

1. The public is longing for empowerment to live well. This is evidenced by a vast movement, especially among the wealthy, for access to spas, wellness clinics, the use of complementary/alternative medicine, and the use of yoga. This is a worldwide movement where countries such as Thailand and India are

positioning themselves to be the future of wellness and medical care with a strong emphasis on wellness.

2. The United States has an army of wellness providers in the form of massage therapists, acupuncturists, herbalists, chiropractors, wellness and holistically-oriented physicians and nurses. However, because of the way funding works, most of these individuals do not focus on promoting wellness, but are focused on promoting care reimbursed by insurance within the existing system; thus they are diverted from their main interest of educating the individual on how to be well.

3. This longing for learning about wellness and how to live well is emphasized continuously on shows such as those by Montel Williams and Oprah Winfrey, and through enormous sales of books by Andrew Weil, Deepak Chopra, and Mehmet Oz, etc. The public longs for this kind of learning.

4. There are demonstration projects. For example, the British Government recently funded a project in Devon with Dr. Michael Dixon and Simon Mills, who have devised a wellness program that gives local primary care physicians funding incentives to invest in wellness, and provides them the freedom to keep for the community any funding not needed for disease-care. It is an inventive system to promote wellness and to reduce the habit of turning to high-tech, higher cost interventions.

5. Many of the components for an American wellness system are available. They must be triggered by certain public policy steps to redirect the way in which cash flows – a way of breaking the iron triangle.

6. We break the iron triangle with a focus on a wellness system designed to move 75 percent of the public (a public that now repeatedly goes to disease experts) into learning wellness practices – how to breathe, how to sleep, how to exercise, and how to live well. It is a conversation about what is **not insurable**. Wellness must be incentivized, but we cannot **insure** well-living. We must figure out from a public policy perspective how to encourage young children in the first grade to breathe deeply, to get enough sleep, and to eat well. For example, rather than immediately resorting to the pharmaceutical Ritalin, we must learn how to incentivize deep breathing and exercise for hyperactive children.

Public Policies

1. The president must use his "pulpit" to preach that health-care reform must start with an individual responsibility to live well using wise habits: enough sleep, simple food, plenty of exercise, and leisure time with family and friends. This seems to be the president's personal lifestyle — focused not on preventing illness, but on wise habits through which we feel good about being alive.

2. We must create a White House Office charged with promoting the habits of wellness in every aspect of American life. Wellness is not only a matter for the health-care system; it must be developed through the engagement of our educational system, our businesses, our environmental awareness, our military families, our veterans services, etc.

3. We must fund demonstration initiatives in local communities, designed to reduce medical expenditures when healthy

lifestyle habits are reinforced at a community level. Howard County, Maryland, currently has such a demonstration project for the uninsured. These demonstrations should provide financial and community-benefit incentives for corporations and local governments to build wellness programs. Most self-insured corporations and local governments and colleges have a financial self-interest in promoting such initiatives. These wellness programs must be incentivized with demonstration funding.

4. Funds provided for disease research must remain level, while additional funds should be used to build and research a wellness model for our society.

5. Wellness must not be insurance-linked. Insurance must be used to tend pathologies when there are recognized ways to help. Tax-exempt savings accounts may incentivize the transition from a disease model to a wellness culture. (Nortin Hadler, at the Medical School at the University of North Carolina, has written widely on this topic.)

6. All current health-care providers must be trained to understand their own bodies, i.e., how to maintain their own wellness. Most health-care workers endure extreme stress and are very vulnerable to chronic illnesses. Like most Americans, health-care workers tend to take a pill in the presence of a headache rather than relieve the stress that generated the headache.

7. This training for health-care workers will effectively enable each of them to become a wellness coach. As health-care workers learn to tend their own wellness, they will become a national army of wellness educators able to instruct those who come to them, guiding them to maximize wellness and deal effectively with symptoms before their symptoms become pathologies.

8. Individuals and families must learn to be their own primary care providers. Our disease-oriented system will become more efficient as people learn how to function with day-to-day symptoms and to manage chronic disorders, and thus move out of this disease system. Thus demand for disease-care services will decrease, making access and funding available for those who do need immediate care for a pathology.

9. The United States must fund the development of a series of wellness universities (such as Tai Sophia) to train wellness educators for our schools and our communities.

APPENDIX C

A Strategic Plan *for* a Wellness Culture

Samueli Institute is a non-profit research organization supporting the scientific investigation of healing and its role in medicine and health care. Founded in 2001 by Henry and Susan Samueli, the Institute is advancing the science of healing worldwide. Samueli Institute's focus includes complementary, alternative and integrative medicine, optimal healing environments, relationship-centered care, the role of the mind and lifestyle in healing, health-care policy research, and military and veterans health research.

An overarching program of the Institute is the Wellness Initiative for the Nation (WIN), devised to proactively prevent disease and illness, promote health and productivity, and create well-being and flourishing for the people of America. The WIN addresses strategies for creating health, saving costs, and enhancing wellness through a concerted focus on self-care, core lifestyle change, and integrative health-care practices.

For a document about WIN that provides a precise national strategy with extensive citations, visit the Samueli website at www.siib.org.

Resources

Websites

www.siib.org. Information about WIN (Wellness Initiative for the Nation), a project that promotes health and productivity, creating well-being while saving costs, is available at the Samueli Institute website.

www.tedxmidatlantic.com. Videos of speakers at TED events are available at this website, including Robert Duggan's talk at the November 5, 2009 TEDx event in Baltimore.

www.help.senate.gov/hearings. Videos and transcripts of testimony before the US Senate Committee on Health, Education, Labor, & Pensions (HELP) are available on the HELP website, including Robert Duggan's testimony at the February 23, 2009 hearing titled "Principles of Integrative Care: A Path to Health Care Reform," and the testimony of Catherine M. Baase, MD, Global Director of Health Services for the Dow Chemical Company, titled "Principles of Integrated Health: A Path to Health Care Reform."

www.iom.edu. Reports from the Institute of Medicine (IOM) regarding integrative care, including "Insuring America's Health: Principles and Recommendations," are available at the IOM website.

www.nationalhealthfreedom.org. With the vision of "a healthy nation, with empowered people, making informed health-care decisions," the National Health Freedom Coalition provides documents, articles, legislation, and more at this website.

www.cmbm.org. The Center for Mind-Body Medicine teaches scientifically-validated mind-body medicine techniques that enhance each person's capacity for self-awareness and self-care. Its website includes information about professional training opportunities, self-care techniques, research, and more.

www.sustaincare.net. The SustainCare Community Interest project supports the goal of "learning to look after ourselves and our families in ways that make sense and do not cost the earth." Based in Exeter, England, SustainCare creates classes, community events, and website materials that enable self-care.

www.tai.edu. Tai Sophia Institute, an accredited graduate school, offers master's degrees in Acupuncture, Health and Wellness Coaching, Transformative Leadership and Social Change, Nutrition and Integrative Health, Therapeutic Herbalism, Oriental Medicine, as well as graduate certificates in related studies. Its website includes information about these programs and other resources for learning, healing, and wellness.

www.wisdomwell.info. A family acupuncture and wellness center, WisdomWell shares these simple yet powerful philosophies: The body is wise; you can be your best "primary care provider"; nature is one of our greatest teachers; wellness is about the day-to-day and is best achieved in community. WisdomWell's services feature acupuncture, herbalism and nutrition, massage, individual yoga, craniosacral therapy, counseling and coaching, and wellness consulting.

Books

Shannon Brownlee, *Overtreated: Why Too Much Medicine is Making Us Sicker and Poorer* (Bloomsbury Press, 2008).

Daniel Callahan, *The Troubled Dream of Life: In Search of Peaceful Death* (Georgetown University Press, 2000).

David Cayley, *Ivan Illich in Conversation* (House of Anansi Press, 1992).

Deepak Chopra, *Perfect Health: The Complete Mind/Body Guide* (Harmony Books, revised and updated edition, 2001).

Deepak Chopra, *Reinventing the Body, Resurrecting the Soul: How to Create a New You* (Three Rivers Press, reprint edition, 2010).

Dianne Connelly, *Medicine Words: Language of Love for the Treatment Room of Life* (WisdomWell Press, 2009). *All Sickness is Home Sickness* (WisdomWell Press, 1993).

Larry Dossey, *The Extraordinary Healing Power of Ordinary Things: Fourteen Natural Steps to Health and Happiness* (Three Rivers Press, 2007).

Robert M. Duggan, *Common Sense for the Healing Arts* (Tai Sophia Press, 2003).

James S. Gordon, *Manifesto for a New Medicine: Your Guide to Healing Partnerships and the Wise Use of Alternative Therapies* (Da Capo Press, 1997).

Nortin M. Hadler, *The Last Well Person: How to Stay Well Despite the Health-care System* (McGill-Queens University Press, 2004).

Nortin M. Hadler, *Stabbed in the Back: Confronting Back Pain in an Overtreated Society* (University of North Carolina Press, 2009).

Nortin M. Hadler, *Worried Sick: A Prescription for Health in an Overtreated America* (University of North Carolina Press, 2008).

Jonathan Haidt, *The Happiness Hypothesis: Finding Modern Truth in Ancient Wisdom* (Basic Books, 2006).

Hastings Center, *From Birth to Death and Bench to Clinic: The Hastings Center Bioethics Briefing Book for Journalists, Policymakers, and Campaigns* (Garrison, NY: The Hastings Center, 2008).

Ivan Illich, *Limits to Medicine: Medical Nemesis, The Expropriation of Health* (Marion Boyars Publishers, 2000).

Bill Moyers, *Healing and the Mind,* Companion Volume to Bill Moyers' PBS TV Series (Main Street Books, 1995).

Dean Ornish, *Dr. Dean Ornish's Program for Reversing Heart Disease: The Only System Scientifically Proven to Reverse Heart Disease Without Drugs or Surgery* (Ivy Books, 1995).

Candace B. Pert, *Molecules Of Emotion: The Science Behind Mind-Body Medicine* (Simon & Schuster, 1999).

Michael Pollan, *The Omnivore's Dilemma: A Natural History of Four Meals* (Penguin, 2007).

Martin E. P. Seligman, *Flourish: A Visionary New Understanding of Happiness and Well-Being* (New York: Free Press, Division of Simon & Schuster, 2011).

Peter M. Senge, C. Otto Scharmer, Joseph Jaworski, Betty Sue Flowers, *Presence: An Exploration of Profound Change in People, Organizations, and Society* (Crown Buisness, 2005).

John Travis and Regina Sara Ryan, *The Wellness Workbook: How to Achieve Enduring Health and Vitality*, 3rd edition (Celestial Arts, 2004).

Andrew Weil, *Eight Weeks to Optimal Health: A Proven Program for Taking Full Advantage of Your Body's Natural Healing Power* (Ballantine Books, 1998).

About the Author

An educator, acupuncturist, and healer for more than 40 years, Bob Duggan is a pioneering leader in the emergence of complementary medicine — now often called integrative medicine — and a ground-breaking voice for wellness in the United States. He is the founder, president emeritus, and a faculty member of the Tai Sophia Institute, the first accredited acupuncture school in America, which today offers many master's-degree and certificate programs in the wellness field. Bob has dedicated his career to working with individuals, corporate and academic leaders, policymakers, and legislators to bring a great diversity of healing options to the American people. In 1972 when Bob started studying acupuncture, it was largely illegal across America. Facing the threat of imprisonment, he played a leading role in paving the path to create certification, licensing, and accreditation, solidifying acupuncture as a profession and bringing it into the mainstream culture. A nationally-recognized thought leader, speaker, and advisor to policymakers and organizations on complementary medicine and wellness, Bob has testified before the Senate Committee on Health, Education, Labor, and Pensions, and has spoken at events sponsored by the National Institutes of Health and the White House Commission on Complementary and Alternative Medicine. Bob holds advanced degrees in philosophy, theology, human relations, inter-cultural communications, canon law, and acupuncture, and has served as a priest in the US and abroad. He earned a master's degree in Human Relations and

Community Studies from New York University and a master's degree in Moral Theology from St. Joseph's Seminary. His master's qualification in Acupuncture is from the College of Traditional Chinese Acupuncture in the United Kingdom. He is a nationally-certified Diplomate of Acupuncture and a licensed acupuncturist in the State of Maryland.

Breaking the Iron Triangle is Bob's second book. He also wrote *Common Sense for the Healing Arts*, a collection of essays offering practical wisdom for living well. In addition to consulting with organizations on wellness and healing, Bob maintains a private practice, working alongside his family at WisdomWell in Columbia, MD, a center for family wellness and a gathering place for community learning.